HOME HEALTH CARE THE EASY WAY
A Step–by–Step Guide
to Caring for a Patient in Your Home

Written by
Diane M. Burgan
with
Lois V. Seamans, R.N.,B.S.
Illustrations by Linda Riek

Creative Opportunities, Orangevale, California

Home Health Care The Easy Way
A Step–by–Step Guide
to Caring for a Patient in Your Home.
By
Diane M. Burgan
with
Lois Seamans, R.N., B.S.

Published by Creative Opportunities Publishing Company
P.O. Box 2461
Orangevale, CA 95662 U.S.A.

Publisher's Cataloging-in-Publication

Burgan, Diane M.
    Home health care the easy way : a step-by-step guide to caring for a patient in your home / written by Diane M. Burgan with Lois V. Seamans ; illustrations by Linda Riek.
    -- 1st ed.
    p. cm.
    Includes index.
    Preassigned LCCN: 97-92465
    ISBN: 0-9660704-0-2

    1. Home nursing--Popular works. 2. Caregivers. 3. Aged--Home care--Handbooks, manuals, etc.   I. Seamans, Lois V.
II. Riek, Linda. III. Title.

RT61.B87 1998   649.8
                                 QBI98-560

DEDICATION

This book is dedicated to my husband, Darrell Fronczek and the memory of his parents, Louis & Mary Fronczek.

ACKNOWLEDGEMENT

A heartfelt "thank you" is sent to the following individuals:my sister-in-law, Lois Seamans, for her professional expertise in the area of nursing and enthusiasm for this book. Kit Moser (of the infamous writing team, "Spangenburg & Moser")for her technical help, professional editing skills and constant encouragement, and Kim DeFilippis, friend and confidante. Grazie Mille!

WARNING-DISCLAIMER

TABLE OF CONTENTS

———

CHAPTER I
HOME HEALTH CARE INDUSTRY : BUYER BEWARE

The Labor Department states that home health care is now the nation's fastest growing industry and will continue to have the largest growth of any U.S. industry through the year 2005. There are many reasons for this tremendous explosion of growth. The cost of in-home care is far less than both hospital care and nursing home care combined. Sick people seem to thrive better in a familiar environment where they feel most comfortable. They don't get as depressed and the care they receive is more personal because it is one on one. Medicare pays for limited home care, as do the Medicaid, Older Americans Act and Social Services Block Grant programs.

Another reason for this growth is that more and more medical insurers are endorsing and providing some coverage for home health care professionals. But not all have come around. Check your policy carefully to see if any coverage is offered for in-home care by professionals. If you qualify for outside help, take advantage of it even if it is for just a few hours a day. The responsibility of round-the-clock care of another person will be extremely difficult, if not impossible without some relief. With or without insurance coverage, you may still want to hire your own outside workers either through an agency or on your own.

Unfortunately, growth can mean problems and the rapid rise in home health care, combined with loose licensing laws and lax oversight has meant an increase in fraud, theft and abuse of the elderly.This year, Medicare and Medicaid, the government insurance programs for the elderly, poor and disabled, will lose an estimated $2.2 billion to fraudulent home-care providers. It is a poorly regulated business and the buyer should "beware." Federal and state rules that govern nursing homes don't apply in private homes.

Each day, millions of elderly Americans open their doors to people hired to take care of them and instead find themselves victimized by scam artists. Part of the problem is that the concept of home health care is not what it used to be. The definitions of home care and the people who provide it have blurred. Today patients can get personal care attendants, home health aides, nurses and various therapists. These individuals may be responsible for everything from housekeeping to intravenous drug therapy. Many people assume that agencies will do a background check on their workers before they're hired. In fact, many don't do any kind of a check and rely on workers to freely disclose negative information , including the existence of criminal records.

The National Association of Home Care, the largest home care industry group, represents 6,000 of the more than 17,000 home care agencies. They currently estimate that as many as 7 million people receive home health care through agencies or private arrangements. Most provide no assurances that their care givers are not incompetant or convicted criminals. Both types can easily slip into the home care business and reports of abuse and neglect are rising at an alarming rate. The N.A.H.C. wants to see stricter, uniform training along with standard licensing and screening procedures for workers–all deemed necessary to weed out bad providers.

Most states have no established channel for complaints of abuse, neglect and theft in home care settings. The problems run the circular path between nursing home regulators, adult protective services and the local police. And worse, the elderly who are abused or stolen from, tend not to report the crime for fear they will be sent to a nursing home . If they do speak up, it's usually to the agency who hired the abusive workers in the first place. And nobody seems to be watching the agencies. So how *do* you find a quality home health care agency? Should you just hire workers on your own?

There is no right answer. If you hire privately, you must take all responsibility as an employer–screening candidates, paying taxes, ensuring proper supervision. In some states, home care rules don't apply to independent hires. With agency hires, there's often more state oversight and the company bears some responsibility for its workers screening and conduct. But even that's not a guarantee.

Although most states don't require criminal background checks , some home care agencies will do them anyway. These background checks don't guarantee good care, and the quality can vary tremendously from one agency to another. Find out what's being checked and who's doing the checking. You can also do your own background checks including fingerprinting potential employees to check for criminal records. Forms must be signed by the applicant giving you authorization to see these records. (See Appendix B)

If that seems like too much work, there are companies for hire whose sole purpose is to do background checks. Make up your own questionnaire for potential employees. You should check references, as many as possible. Be on the lookout for phony places of employment. Make sure the companies really exist and the references really worked there at one time.

No matter which way you decide to go, be wary of giving any care giver access to a patient's funds–don't write blank checks, and keep a close eye on credit card statements and bank statements. Mailing sensitive financial statements to a third party is an even better option. Generally speaking, no care giver, unless bonded, should deal with a patient's finances.

Make sure care is monitored by a relative or friend. Look for signs of physical abuse: unexplained bumps or bruises. Psychological abuse is more difficult to spot, but if a patient becomes withdrawn or starts changing established routines, a closer look may be warranted. Agencies should document training for care givers.

For nurses, check with the state's licensing authorities to make sure that the person's license is in good order. Some states require aides to pass a state-administered test. Find out if your state lists certified aides, as well as any disciplinary actions, on a registry.

Ask for referrals from as many people as you can. Your medical doctor should be aware of an agency in your area. Also, the hospital discharge planner is another good source for referrals. But if any of these people say they aren't familiar with these services, you will have to do some research. Use the Yellow Pages. Look under *home health care or nursing.* [**Note:** Beware of any organization calling itself a "registry" and not a home health agency. A "registry" doesn't need a license but often is listed under " Home Health Services" in the Yellow Pages and can be recommended by local hospitals.]

The community liaison or spokesperson for a home health care agency will visit nursing homes, doctors offices, insurance companies and anyone else who would benefit from having information about the services the agency provides. If someone is having difficulty with the home care service, the liaison steps in and tries to resolve the problem. Home health care agencies want your business and should not object to your asking numerous questions about their service.

Qualify the agencies to make sure they will not only meet the patient's needs but will only send competent, honest workers to your house. And you do that by asking lots of questions. Here are a few that should be asked of any health care provider:

1. Is the agency a **Medicare** provider? Even if the patient is not a medicare patient, Medicare is regulated by certain federal guidelines, called Title 22. These

guidelines are very specific about the qualifications of the employees and what kinds of care they can provide. If the agency is not a Medicare provider that doesn't mean they're not a good agency. It's just something for you to take into consideration as you make your decision.

2. Is the agency licensed by the state? If so, they are also governed by state rules and regulations.

3. Are they accredited by the Joint Commission Accreditation Health Care Organizations (J.A.C.O.) or the National League for Nursing ? This is a service conducted by nonprofit professional   organizations. Accreditation means the agency has met basic standards, especially in the area of personnel requirements, supervision and accountability. Participation by the health care agencies is voluntary. Just because the agency is not accredited doesn't mean it's not a good agency.

4. Are all agency employees and subcontractors they may hire covered by workers compensation insurance? Are they bonded? Does the agency do background checks?

The next step is to supply the agency with all the necessary information on the patient: the medical history, therapy needs, medication needs, doctors name etc. This is also where insurance is discussed.

In order to get skilled care paid for by third–party reimbursement, you need a doctor's order. **Medicare A** is standard medicare; anyone 65 or over who has worked qualifies. **Medicare B** is extra coverage that you can buy. The agency should do the billing for you–it's one of the advantages of hiring one. They will help you determine who will be the primary insurance carrier and what types of services will be billed to it.The best–case scenario is to have both Medicare and private insurance. Medicare provides for intermittant care, not continuous care. A nurse comes in, does the task and leaves or a therapist comes in, does the therapy and leaves. Medicare also does pay for some education. An agency can send a nurse to the home to teach you how to do the task.

Most health care agencies will do a free assessment of the patient and then bill Medicare for the service. If Medicare won't pay, make sure you won't be charged.

First, a nurse is sent in to evaluate the patient and determine the kinds of services needed. Then the agency approaches the patient's doctor. The agency needs to work hand-in-hand with the doctor, because all third party reimbursement is based on doctor's orders. The agency then develops a plan of care or treatment for the doctor's approval and signature. This plan has to be reviewed on a continuing basis, every 60 days or so.

If you have no insurance and don't qualify for Medicare,a good agency will direct you to other resources available. Or, you can pay the agency directly. The average hourly rate for home health aides, which is the least skilled care available, is $14.00 an hour. Live-in rates run approximately $130.00 to $160.00 per 24 hour period. These rates include insurance and social security taxes for the worker, which the agency pays.

The agency hires or subcontracts many different workers. Not everybody needs to be an R.N. to care for the patient. Sometimes all that's needed is help with simple tasks–house cleaning and cooking for instance. A **certified nursing assistant** or **nonskilled provider** has completed the basic CPR course, has first aid knowledge and has usually completed some kind of an assistant program that usually lasts 18 weeks. Some convalescent homes offer the training free of charge and in return get six months of service when the students get their certificates. These workers cannot give medications or change dressings. They can do light housework,feed, bathe and clean up the patient. Their duties also include simply helping the patient to move from one place to another in the home.

A *licensed practical nurse or licensed vocational nurse (LPN or LVN)* goes through an 18–month or two–year program, get practical experience in a hospital as well as classroom schooling. They receive training at a higher technical level and are allowed to perform more of the procedures that the aides cannot, such as, give medications, change dressings and do an assessment of the patient. They also can take the state license exam that registered nurses take.

A *registered nurse* can go through either a two–year associates degree program or a four–year bachelor's program. No matter what program they go through, they take the same state exam and are considered to be equally qualified no matter what degree they possess.

An agency will often recruit their staff through newspaper ads, medical journals and word of mouth before hiring. They hire part–time and full–time workers. Most people go into nursing for the flexible hours.

The agency supervises its employees' work and monitors the quality of their performance. The registered nurse usually becomes the case manager and acts in a more supervisory position. This is the person who goes into the home and does the assessment and returns for a follow–up visit to see how the patient is responding to the treatment prescribed.

Before hiring, a good agency will check out the references and test the skills of their prospective employees, including a written exam. Once hired, the agency will review all the paperwork their employees are required to complete regarding the patient. A supervisor will also do a home visit and talk to the families and, if they can, to the patient, to make sure things are working out well. There also is a performance review for agency workers, depending on the number of hours they work. Usually, after 60 hours worked or 120 hours, a supervisor goes to the home and watches the employee perform the tasks required. A good question to ask the agency: "Do you have a nursing supervisor who comes out and evaluates the performance of the worker and how often do you do this?"

The doctor will order all medical equipment, based on the home assessment and his or her own recommendations. Again, this medical order from a licensed physician is necessary to get third party reimbursement.

Many home health care agencies require money up front before services begin. There can be a discrepancy between agencies on this matter, so be sure to ask!

According to the National Association for Home Care, home care consumers (clients) have a right to be notified in writing of their rights and obligations before treatment is begun. The client's family or guardian may exercise the client's rights when the client has been judged incompetent. Home care providers have an obligation to protect and promote the rights of their clients. Clients have the right:

- to have relationships with home care providers that are based on honesty and ethical standards of conduct;

- to be informed of the procedure they can follow to lodge complaints with the home care provider about the care that is, or fails to be, furnished, and regarding a lack of respect for property;

- to know about the disposition of such complaints;

- to voice their grievances without fear of discrimination or reprisal for having done so;

- to be advised of the telephone number and hours of operation of the state's home health "hot line."

Clients also have the right:

- to be notified in writing of the care that is to be furnished, the types (disciplines) of the caregivers who will furnish the care and the frequency of the visits that are proposed to be furnished;

- to be advised of any change in the plan of care before the change is made;

- to participate in the planning of the care and in planning changes in the care, and to be advised that they have the right to do so; and

- to refuse services or request a change in caregiver without fear of reprisal or discrimination.

Regarding financial information, clients have the right:

- to be informed of the extent to which payment may be expected from Medicare, Medicaid or any other payor known to the home care provider;

- to be informed of the charges that will not be covered by Medicare;

- to be informed of the charges for which the client may be liable;

- to receive this information, orally and in writing, within 15 working days of the date the home care provider becomes aware of any changes in charges; and

- to have access, upon request, to all bills for service the client has received regardless of whatever they are paid out-of-pocket or by another party.

CHAPTER II
PLANNING THE HOME
HEALTH CARE ROOM

A little bit of planning goes a long way. If the patient is in the hospital, insist on knowing exactly when he will be discharged to your care. This will allow you to visit a few health supply stores to rent and/or buy the equipment needed to furnish the *care room.*

Find out what the guidelines are for Medicare and what items will be covered. And be sure to consult the discharging doctor. Most items ordered by the physician by writing a prescription are covered by Medicare.

Examine your home and choose a room (not necessarily the bedroom) best suited to accomodate the patient. Ideally, the room should have easy access to the care giver and all visitors during the day, yet not be isolated at night. It should be close to a bathroom, and have windows with a view. When patients are bedridden, if they can feel a cool breeze on their face and watch the seasons change, they are less likely to feel isolated and depressed.

The room should be large enough to accomodate both a bed and sitting area for visitors. Stairs should be avoided at all costs. A patient who is physically challenged either through age or illness does not need the added physical trial of stairs. Also, the caregiver does not need the added challenge of stairs, every time the call bell rings.

Avoid loose rugs on the floor which might cause tripping or slipping. Pay attention to doorknobs. They can become frustrating barriers for weak and arthritic hands. Replace slippery knobs with larger, textured ones or glue covers of heavy fabric on them.

Color can play a big role in mood. Decorate with warm, light colors to brighten and cheer the patient and visitors. Cover any glares or extreme light coming from the windows with sheer curtains or blinds. Install a night light to illuminate the path to the bathroom.

Often the elderly patient's internal temperature-control mechanism is not as adaptable as the rest of the family's. Chilling the house at night should be avoided. A person confined to the bed is more comfortable when there is no sweating from excessive heat. Try to find a household temperature that works for all members of the household.

The bedside table functions as a mini-convenience store for the bedridden and should be large enough to accomodate bottles of medicine, snacks, books, and other items of diversion.

There are many items that can be added to the room to help the patient stay in touch with day–in and day–out reality. A telephone provides security and enjoyment for the patient unable to get out and visit with friends and family. You might consider getting a long extension cord instead of a fixed installation put in by the telephone company. Or consider a cordless phone so the patient can easily walk around the room.

A colorful calendar posted on the wall keeps track of days, seasons, and events. Use a calendar that requires a page to be torn off. It can be a daily activity to tear the page off and face the new day.

Keep a television in the room in a comfortable viewing position with the remote control easily accessible. But don't let it take over. Although television is a good distractor for the elderly and bedridden, it does not stimulate any mental or physical activity. Make sure elderly patients do not spend the entire day watching soap operas and game shows. Keep them busy, moving and alert.

Movement of the joints, jogging of the memory and the maintenance of other necessary bodily functions are hindered by inactivity. Music is a nice alternative. Don't forget a radio or portable CD /tape player that can be controlled by the patient. A clock with a large face and bold numerals is very useful. Make sure it doesn't have a loud, irritating tick that disturbs light sleepers.

Some bedridden patients tend to disregard personal appearance and hygiene. Avoid unwashed hair, untrimmed nails and sloppy clothes. Keep the pressure on for good grooming, even if company isn't coming on that day. A full–length mirror can help someone with poor eyesight or dimmed memory with dressing.

Flowers and plants add a feeling of life to a room and a sense of responsibility to the caretaker of the plants. Depending on your patient's interests and abilities, there are many variables that can be added for interest: bright mobiles, reading materials, pictures, and various crafts to be worked on.

No matter how comfortable and attractive the patient's room, over time, the walls will tend to close in and the bed becomes a prison. Even with a nice window, much of what is outside will remain unseen. Many bedridden patients can be helped into a wheelchair and taken outside to feel the breeze on their face. Do this as often as possible–it can truly lift the spirits! Also, try keeping a chair by the bed that the patient can be easily helped into.

Safety within the home requires preparation. Falls account for approximately 80% of the deaths of the elderly. Deaths from falls in individuals 75 years of age and above are almost four times as high as those between 65 and 74. We use the word "accidents" to describe these falls but in fact they usually occur because of carelessness.

The mobility of the home health care patient, especially the elderly, is determined by many factors. Accordingly, they may require a wheelchair, walker, or cane. Some patients will be able to move about the house but before they do, check the placement or furniture and floor coverings. Throw rugs on slippery floors are an accident waiting to happen. A sharp table edge or unsteady plant should be removed. If there are children in the house, establish firm rules about toys or clothes being left on the floor. Small children and animals can trip an unsuspecting, unsteady patient.

Do a walk–through of your home and hunt for potential hazards such as loose floor coverings, lamp cords that cross traffic lanes, small dark obstacles such as sewing baskets or piles of books, poorly lit stairs, absence of handrails, etc.

The bathroom deserves special attention; it is often the source of unnecessary accidents. Every effort should be made to maximize the efficiency and safety of this room. Install antiskid strips in the bathtub and grab bars on the wall. Large, flat mats with nonskid backing will usually prevent slipping. Many toilets are low and difficult for an elderly or handicapped person to sit down on and get back up. You can purchase a relatively inexpensive raised toilet seat attachment that slips on and off a regular toilet bowl and places the seat at a comfortable position. When you use such devices, make sure the original paper holder is in a new, convenient position.

Scalding water accidents can be greatly reduced by keeping the household hot water at a temperature no greater than 120 Fahrenheit. Most elderly patients get accidently scalded because their reflexes are not fast enough or they are not agile enough to turn the water off quickly.

Check for portable heaters that are too close to curtains and towels,electrical appliances too close to water,breakable glass containers, razors and sharp scissors. Search out and store separately cleaning solutions and toiletries that might be confused with medicines by those with failing eyesight.

How much care and attention should be giving to making the home environment stress and accident free? Compromises will have to be made for few homes can be modified to one's complete satisfaction. Work on those items that will be most beneficial with the least possible cost. Even the most favorable physical arrangements will not erase all difficulties. Space will have to be shared by the able-bodied and the not-so-able. Don't compromise your lifestyle and particularly that of your children.

CHAPTER III
COPING WITH THE STRESS

Caring for a patient at home means a change in the family structure and that change will be felt throughout the entire family. Each member must find a way to adjust to the situation and cope with the stresses that change creates.

Solitude, or quality time away from your task as caregiver is necessary for your sanity. Build some free time into your schedule every day.Perhaps midmorning would be a good time for a break or late evening. When you feel the need, retreat to your bedroom to have some free time to talk with friends on the phone, read, write, watch TV or just relax. If you have children, they also should not be denied their normal activities. Everyone is entitled to periods of solitude.

Sharing the bathroom with yet another family member can be extremely difficult. Try to establish rules and a schedule to remove bottlenecks. Extra towels and racks can be installed and assigned to each member of the family. Some functions, such as grooming, or shaving with an electric shaver, can be moved to the bedroom. Try to think of other tricks to keep the traffic moving. Improving the environment often times reduces the stress that can occur when you share your home with the home care patient.

Remember, coping is a two pronged process. You must have the ability to control not only yourself but those around you as well. In coping with the aging home care patient, it is important to understand the psychodynamics of aging; you must know what old age is and what to expect from it.

Gerontologists have catalogued the significant characteristics associated with old age. This often includes slowness of thinking, mild impairment of recent memory, reduction in enthusiasm, tendency towards depression, narcissism, change in sleep patterns, an increase in daytime naps, and increased attention to one's bowels and other bodily functions. Aging varies from individual to individual and you may not see all of these signs at once.

There are many seniors who remain enthusiastic, productive and mobile well past their peers.

If you are caring for an aging patient, help him to stay in touch with reality. Talk about current events. Use newspapers and the television to keep them aware of the time, date, and daily routines. Sensory deprivation is often the source of confusion and abnormal behavior. When people are confined to small spaces, such as their bedrooms, they experience greater sensory deprivation. Don't let an elderly patient hibernate! Try not to let the elderly patient fall into the trap of acting fragile or incompetent. The more you do, the less they will be able to do and soon you will find yourself doing everything such as buttoning, cutting meat and picking up small things. Help when necessary but try not to patronize and pamper.

When the elderly patient becomes depressed because of a painful terminal illness or seemingly irreparable loss, thoughts of suicide suddenly become common. Many elderly talk about suicide but do nothing about it. Then there are those who never say a word but do commit the act. Even professionals have difficulty in evaluating the signals of suicide. Fortunately, many suicide attempts by the elderly are unsuccessful and the underlying causes discovered and treated. For others, it is their last act of self-determination.

You are not alone in your predicament of caring for a sick or elderly patient, often one's own parent. Many agencies listed in the Yellow Pages under Social Services are willing to help you in a variety of ways. And if they can't, they are the first to refer you to one that can.

Start with your patient's primary care physician. Many hospitals have social service departments that can help you whether or not your patient was recently hospitalized. Your community church can also be an excellent referral source. There are senior citizen centers in most communities that offer a healthy diversion to the elderly. Check the heading Office on Aging in the telephone directory or under local governmental services. If financial aid is required call the local Social Security office first and then the county welfare department. Remember, these agencies want you; they need you to stay in business. Contacting an agency to help you is one of the smartest things you can do to help cope with the awesome responsibility of caring for a sick or elderly patient in your home. (See Appendix A:)

CHAPTER IV
THE CHANGING FACE OF MANAGED CARE

Health care in America has become a hodge-podge of HMOs, PPOs and IPAs. Confused? You're not the only one. If the transformation of the health care industry doesn't interest you, it should. From gag rules for doctors, restrictions on prescription drugs and even limitations on treatment that are characteristic of managed care health plans, what you don't know can seriously affect your health or the health of your home care patient.

In the 1980's, one reaction to skyrocketing medical costs was Medicare's DRGs (diagnosis-related groupings that set standard payments for particular diagnoses). Along with difficult labor–management negotiations, the end result was health coverage takebacks, including more deductibles and higher co-payments.

President Clinton pushed hard for national health care reform but partisan politics and a barrage of misinformation effectively thwarted his efforts. Instead, the private health care industry went ahead and implemented its own approach to cost savings: managed care.

"Managed Care" says it all: some one or some group manages your health care. To some supporters, managed care plans carefully coordinate each patient's medical care, promote preventive medicine and carefully monitor quality. Detractors say managed care is nothing more than a bureaucratic system that diminishes choice for consumers and forces doctors to place saving money before saving lives.

Under the current fee–for–service arrangement, the patient incurs expenses for health care from doctors that he or she generally selects. The doctor or other provider is then reimbursed for covered services in part by the insurer and in part by the patient, who is responsible for the balance not covered by the insurance company. There is no mechanism in this fee-for-service arrangement to coordinate the care the patient gets from the doctor.

Managed–care arrangements often include a broad and continually changing array of health plans that try to control the cost and quality of care by coordinating the medical services of each patient. Managed care plans include a variety of health maintenance organizations (HMOs), preffered provider organizations (PPOs) and independent practice associations (IPAs).

In typical managed care or prepaid health care arrangements, the managed health care company pays doctors, medical groups and some hospitals a set monthly fee for every "subscriber" or member assigned to their practices. The member agrees to use the health company's providers for all covered health care services. The company then provides comprehensive and preventive health care benefits and agrees to provide all covered services for a set price, the per person premium fee that each member pays (or the employer pays on the member's behalf). Consumers may have to pay additional fees or co-payments for office visits and other services The high mark of managed care is that the company organizes the delivery of your care through an infrastructure it has built among its providers thus ensuring low costs and quality of care.

Managed care plans, like HMOs, usually have a primary care physician whom the member selects, who is responsible for coordinating the patient's care. HMO members must get a referral from the primary care physician before they can see a specialist.

Critics view the role of the primary care physician as that of a "gatekeeper" and an arrangement that is restrictive to patient care. A healthy bottom line depends on keeping costs to a minimum and that means discouraging extensive and expensive medical tests and too many office visits and denying referrals to specialists. Supporters say that when clinical decision making is driven by quality and the desire to prevent illness and disease, this process is the only way to hold down health care costs that have gotten out of control.

The so called "gag rules" that doctors who work for managed care organizations find in their contracts when they sign on with an HMO do nothing to change the perception that HMOs are only about making money not health care. Many doctors who object to gag rules (restrictions on how much the attending physician can tell the patient about tests available and other pertinent information relating to their illness) often find themselves relieved of duty with their contract terminated by the HMO. In fact, many doctors believe the gag rules are in place to hide the fact that doctors often are offered bribes to minimize care.

There is also the problem of "drug formularies"–plans created by health care systems to put certain medications out of reach of patients and physicians. Some plans use incentives or pressure to keep physicians from prescribing nonformulary drugs. Nonlisted medication is either not reimbursed or is subject to a co-pay.

It looks like managed care is here to stay. But the exposure of the horror stories of some patients being denied specialty care, or denied certain extensive testing procedures that would have caught disease sooner, has cast a spotlight on a serious problem. Consumer organizations have already started to rally forth to make sure patient protection plans are in place. In the meantime, you can ask questions before choosing a managed care organization. Here are some terms you need to be familiar with:

HMO (Health Maintenance Organization): An organization that offers comprehensive health benefits to members who prepay a fixed monthly premium. The HMO can be a group model HMO, which contracts with independent medical groups that agree to provide all covered services for the HMO enrollees. Or the HMO can be a staff-model HMO, which employs salaried physicians who provide care only to the HMO enrollees.

PPO (Preferred Provider Organization): The PPO establishes a network of independent physicians who sign a contract to provide covered services for a discounted fee.

IPA (Independent Practice Association): A model of HMO in which individual doctors, who practice in their own offices, sign a contract to provide covered services to enrollees of an HMO. The doctors either sign independently or through a legal entity that negotiates for them. IPA doctors are free to take patients outside of HMO plans or to contract with other HMOs.

POS (Point of Service) This is an option offered by any model HMO. Under the POS option, the patient may choose to obtain covered services from a doctor outside of the HMO network but generally may have to pay more.

NCQA (National Committee for Quality Assurance) An independent, nonprofit organization that accredits HMOs and assesses and reports on health plan quality. The NCQA provides health plan information to consumers free of charge. The NCQA has reviewed 181 of the nation's 547 HMOs, accredited 153 and denied 24.

CHAPTER V
WHO PAYS FOR HEALTH CARE?

The numbers can be mind numbing for health care–as much as $27,000 for a two week stay in a hospital. Along with that add miscellaneous bills for routine medications, $1,700 a year; rehabilitation, $8,500 for a month; and a whopping $30,000 a year for various home care services and $50,000 a year for nursing homes. Who is going to pay for all of that?

In the best of both worlds, public and private insurance programs would unite to pay for this health care. But the reality is that they only cover a portion of it, often times leading to financial ruin for the families. For example, your parents have too little insurance leaving them exposed to enormous financial risk. At the same time, too much insurance means unnecessary payments for premiums and delays for payment if the plans overlap. Now is the time to act on insurance; a parent may become ineligible for certain kinds of insurance as he grows older or if he is diagnosed with a serious illness.

The number one concern on most people's minds is usually long term care, either extended nursing home care or home health care. Hospital stays and doctor bills are largely covered by Medicare and other health insurance policies, but long term care is not. If your parent is still relatively healthy, he should consider long-term health insurance. Speak with a lawyer about how to plan for Medicaid.

Medicare is federal health insurance for people over age 65 and certain disabled individuals under 65. Most individuals over 65 who have been employed or married or widowed from someone who was employed, are eligible for Medicare.

If you are receiving social security payments, you will automatically get a Medicare card at age 65. The enrollment period begins three months before a 65th. birthday and ends four months after. If you miss enrollment during this time it can mean unnecessary delays in payment and possible penalties.

There are two parts to Medicare: Part A is hospital insurance which includes most hospital bills and a limited amount of nursing care. Part B covers medical bills, including medical equipment, doctor's fees, diagnostic tests, outpatient care and some medications. Part B is optional but everyone is automatically enrolled when they become entitled to Part A. If the coverage for Part B is deemed unnecessary (another insurance policy covers the same thing), contact the local social security office to cancel the coverage.

Medicare keeps costs under control by determining in advance what it will pay for each medical procedure. If a doctor accepts this assigned fee as full payment for a given service, the patient pays only the yearly premium ($42.50 a month in 1996), the deductible ($100 in 1996) and the 20 percent co-payment. If the doctor does not accept the fee, then the patient pays the co-payment *plus* the difference between Medicare's approved fee and the doctor's fee. The annual deductible must be met before payments begin.

There is a program in place, *The Qualified Medicare Beneficiary Program (QMB),* that is available for people with incomes at or below the national poverty level, and with limited assets. The state pays Medicare premiums, deductibles and most co-payments. *The Specified Low-Income Medicare Beneficiary Program (SLMB)* is for people whose incomes are up to 10 percent above the national poverty level. The state pays just the Medicare Part B premium.

Medigap refers to private insurance that fills some of the holes in Medicare coverage. It is supplemental insurance intended to pay the cost of premiums, co-payments, deductibles and doctor's bills that exceed Medicare's approved charges. It is highly recommended for most people but isn't necessarily a good choice for anyone who is close to the financial eligibility limits for Medicaid or for someone who is enrolled in a managed care plan or group plan that already provides ample coverage.

Medigap insurance should be purchased within six months of enrolling in Medicare Part B. Coverage cannot be denied during this window of opportunity because of existing medical problems. After this six month period, however, insurance companies can increase prices and attach an array of conditions to the policy.

Most states limit Medigap insurance to ten standard plans that range from Plan A– which is available in all states–through plan J, a much more comprehensive and expensive plan. Any policy should be read carefully to understand what is covered and what exclusions or restrictions exist. Insurance companies are required to provide a clearly worded summary.

Shop around, look for the best price and service you can find and don't compare apples to oranges when it comes to insurance policies. Here are some guidlines for people buying Medigap policies, courtesy of the National Association of Insurance Commissioners and the Health Care Financing Administration:

- Don't duplicate coverage by buying more policies than you need. It's expensive, unnecessary and usually prohibited.

- If you are replacing an existing policy, your parent must be given credit for time spent under the old policy if there are any preexisting conditions or restrictions that apply under a new policy. Never cancel an old policy unless you're absolutely sure that you want the new one!

- Buyer Beware: Know the company you're doing business with. Call the state insurance company and make sure the company or agent is licensed. If you are told that a policy is sponsored by a state agency or that an insurance agent is working for the government–hide your money, neither is true.

- Medigap policies are now required by most states to be guaranteed renewable.

Examine the policy for preexisting-condition exclusions. The phrase, "no medical examination required" can be misleading. If your parent has had a health problem rather recently, there might be a six month moratorium on treatments for that particular health condition. Fill in all information *carefully.* If you accidently leave out any medical history on an application, coverage could be refused for a certain length of time for any medical condition you neglected to mention. Worse, a claim could be denied for treatment of an undisclosed condition or your policy cancelled.

LONG TERM CARE

Nursing home care can quickly eat up a family's savings. Home health care costs less but also requires tremendous resources of time and energy to supervise and coordinate. Either way, both can take a tremendous toll on the families involved . Medicare has many restrictions and pays for about two percent of all nursing home costs nationally. Private insurance covers about one percent of the bill. The remainder is paid privately by individuals, and when that money is spent, Medicaid, the government's insurance program for the poor, is left with the bill.

The cost of long–term care quickly drains a person's assets collected over a lifetime. any people who never dreamed they would need it, find themselves on Medicaid, the government's health insurance program for low-income people. Medicaid pays for about half of all nursing home care nationally. Your parent may qualify for Medicaid long before he thinks he does. Contact a lawyer with your parent to find out about protecting their assets before going on Medicaid. Older people can "spend down," or use up their own money to become eligible for Medicaid. The rules are complicated, try to find a lawyer who specializes in Medicaid planning. Or contact the state legal services office or the state bar association about legal aid to the elderly.

Although the cost of long–term care insurance has come down considerably, it's still a luxury item. Long–term care insurance is usally not an option after age 80 or if someone has a diagnosed or debilitating illness. Prices will vary depending on the type of plan and the age of the insured but premiums can range from $3,000 to $8,500. Who should purchase long-term care insurance?

Those with significant assets. The number one reason to purchase long-term care insurance is to protect your assets. If your parent were to become eligible for Medicaid within 12-18 months of entering a nursing home, they should not purchase a policy.

- Ability to pay, approximately $300 to $500 a month. It is suggested that long-term care insurance should not cost more than 5 percent of a person's total income. Inability to pay the premium will only mean a cancelled policy.

- Take a good look at the family tree based on longevity and disease. A person with a family history of heart disease is less likely to need long-term care than say, someone with a family history of Alzheimer's disease.

The state department of insurance can tell you which insurance companies sell long–term care. You can also look into the cost of attaching a rider onto a current health insurance policy. A few progressive states have currently engaged in partnerships between Medicaid and the insurance industry. Under this plan, individuals who purchase long-term care insurance for , say 3 years, can go on Medicaid when their insurance coverage runs out and still protect a portion of their assets.

Here are some features to look for when purchasing long–term care insurance:

- Wide coverage. Be sure coverage includes home care and custodial care--supervision and help with daily living activities, i.e. eating, bathing and other tasks-- in addition to nursing care.

- Limited Restrictions. Make sure coverage is based on need instead of medical necessities. Your parent should be covered immediately when they need help with personal tasks such as eating, bathing, or dressing.

- Appropriate cost reimbursement. It is common for a policy to pay a fixed amount for each day of long-term care, and your parent pays the rest. The cost of home care is assumed to be half of the rate of nursing home care. Therefore, if the rate of a nursing home is $100 a day then $50 a day is appropriate for home care. Figure our your parent's discretionary income after bills. If a daily stay in the region nursing homes is $115 and your parent has $45 a day in extra income, the difference is the amount of coverage needed in a policy. In this case, $70 a day.

- Allowance for inflation. That extra protection of $70 a day might not be worth much in another ten years when your parent needs it. A policy should allow for inflation, 5 percent is a good figure. Or, if your parent will be needing long term care sooner, consider buying a more generous policy up front.

- Waiting Period. Any waiting period less than 30 days will make the policy more expensive. Likewise, a longer waiting period means a cheaper policy. Be careful of policies with a waiting period of over 100 days. It increases the likelyhood that your parent will never use the policy.

- Maximum Stays. Policies that offer unlimited nursing home care are very expensive. Sometimes coverage is offered on a "per-stay" basis. A policy might cover 75 days straight, then require a break of at least 60 days in between, then cover 75 days again. Other policies offer lifetime limits–a set number of days or a dollar amount that will be covered over your parent's lifetime. Try to find a policy with the highest maximum your parent can afford. Always check the limits on both nursing home and home health care. Each one can have a different maximum limit.

- Waivers. Look for a policy that includes a waiver on premium payments while your parent is receiving long-term care.

- Dementia Coverage. Organic diseases of the brain, such as Alzheimer's, are usually covered in long-term care policies. Check to make sure.

- Renewal .Your long-term care policy should include a guarantee of renewal. Nonpayment of premiums should be the only consideration allowed for cancellation.

- Fixed Premiums. Most elderly people live on fixed incomes. A premium that continues to rise over time means your parent might not be able to afford the policy at a time when they need it the most. Once a policy is purchased, a company is permitted to raise premiums only if it does so for all its policyholders.
- A financially strong company. Check *The Insurance Rating Guide* and make sure the company has a high rating. A financially sound company will be better able to absorb errors in underwriting. This field is still relatively young and companies don't have much history upon which to base their assumptions for underwriting policies. *State guaranteed coverage* for when a company defaults usually means higher premiums, and if the company does fail, the coverage offered by the state won't be nearly as generous as the terms of the policy.

Be careful not to buy into the myth that if your parent is receiving Medicaid they will not get good care. In fact, an expensive nursing home is never a guarantee of loving, professional care. Although appearance is important when deciding the kind of service provided–and should be taken into consideration–it is the people who work in the facility who will be taking care of your loved ones.

It is true that many residences that accept Medicaid will admit only a small number of patients receiving assistance. A nursing home with 250 beds may only reserve 10% of those beds for Medicaid patients. Consequently, you need to get your parent's name on a waiting list for the better Medicaid-certified homes. Set aside enough money to admit your parent as a self-paying resident, at least 6 months worth. Once your parent is admitted, she cannot be discharged when she starts to receive Medicaid even if the portion of Medicaid beds are full.

In order to qualify for Medicaid, a single person is permitted to own no more than their house, some personal belongings, a car and a small amount of savings plus money set aside for burial and funeral expenses. These standards will vary depending upon the disability and medical needs of the person applying. Also taken into consideration is what public assistance he is receiving , life insurance policies, etc.

The rules for couples are more generous, probably because a person who continues to live at home needs to have financial support when a mate enters a nursing home.

Remember, each state has its own set of rules and exceptions and workers in the department of social services are not in a position to advise applicants how to get on Medicaid early and protect their assets. In most states, you need to contact the local department of social services or the human resources administration.   Opportunities to protect assets are rapidly changing and may disappear altogether. What was once permitted may not be today.

Pretend you have a crystal ball and try to anticipate the future for your parents. What will their income be like in three years? Five? Ten? What if illness strikes unexpectedly? Are there any free services or tax credits that your parent may qualify for now? Also, if your parents assets are considerable, they can protect some of them from estate and inheritance taxes. Help your parents to create a financial plan with goals and prioriities firmly in place for their golden years. They may decide to change their spending habits, purchase a Medigap policy, rent out a room in the house for income or sell some assets . Review the plan every six months or when something unexpected happens: a divorce, accident, illness, etc.

A final word of caution. Financial planners and advisers are just that–advisers. It is a rare circumstance indeed where a financial planner should be given legal authority to make financial decisions for or on your parent's behalf *without* your parent's (or your) approval.

SECTION II

 The skills and procedures presented in this next section are intended to ease the stress of the day–in, day–out concerns of caring for a sick, elderly or recuperating patient in the home.

In this section, you will learn how to change an occupied bed, give a complete bed bath, do basic massage therapy, aid with range of motion exercises and more.

Each nursing task has been divided into a logical, orderly sequence of actions or steps. The entire set of steps is known as a procedure. In health care institutions, procedures are done according to a standard method. There are several steps that are common to almost all of the procedures in this book.

Delivering health care is a very special job requiring lots of patience, compassion and empathy.

- Health care providers use their helping hands for the patient.
- Health care providers understand that the patient depends on them.
- Health care providers understand that the patient is someone to comfort and help, not someone to argue with.
- Health care providers use their helping hands to help the patient in a respectful, courteous, and attentive manner.

CHAPTER VI: THE BASICS: Safety, Body Mechanics, Lifting

The patient unit consists of all room space, furniture and equipment provided for the patient. This equipment might include:

- Alternating Pressure mattress. A device like an air mattress placed beneath the bedridden or elderly patient. It reduces pressure on the shoulders, heels, and elbows.

- Bed Board. A large board placed beneath the mattress to provide additional support for patients with back muscle or bone problems.

- Bed Cradle. A frame shaped like a barrel cut in half lengthwise used to eliminate pressure and keep bed linens off a part of the patient's body.

- Egg-crate Mattress. Sometimes called egg-shell mattresses. It reduces pressure on the back, shoulders, heels, elbows and bony prominences.

- Lamb's Wool. A wide strip of lamb's hide or synthetic materials used to relieve pressure in the treatment or prevention of bedsores.

- Portable patient lift. Sometimes called mechanical lift and Hoyer lift. A mechanical device used to move the patient from bed to chair and back again, when the patient needs full assistance.

- Specialty bed. Used to eliminate pressure points and prevent bedsores.

- Walker. A supportive device used by the patient for help in walking.

- Wheelchair. A chair with wheels used to transport patients.

Disposable Equipment

- Plastic Gloves

- Urinal

- Bedpan

- Tissues

- Toilet paper

Safety within the patient unit

Patients challenged by illness, disabilities and medication cannot take care of themselves in an emergency and must be protected. Special care must be taken to guard against accidents, prevent fires and other kinds of emergencies.

- Be sure to lock the brakes on the wheelchair when moving patients on or off.
- When you see something on the floor, pick it up. If you see spilled liquid, wipe up the area.
- Know where the fire extinguisher is located and how it is rated. Type A is for paper,wood and trash; Type B is for liquids such as oil or grease; Type C is for electrical fires. Type ABC may be used safely on all three types of fires.
- If smoking is allowed see that ashtrays are provided and used.
- Empty ashtrays only after all smoking materials have been extinguished for a long time.

- A patient who has been given a sedative should <u>not</u> be allowed to smoke or should have someone present.

- If oxygen is in use, <u>smoking is not allowed!</u> Place a "NO SMOKING:OXYGEN IN USE" sign on the door and on the wall over the patient's bed.
- Dirty linen is <u>never</u> placed on the floor or over the bed table. The floor is already dirty and should not be contaminated again with used linen. Use a separate hamper or basket .
- Do not shake or touch dirty linen to your clothing. Germs are spread easily in this kind of environment.

BODY MECHANICS: LIFTING

When an action requires physical effort, try to use larger muscles or groups of muscles whenever possible. Use both hands rather than one hand to pick up a heavy item.

Use good posture. Keep your back straight and your knees bent with your weight evenly balanced on both feet. Always <u>face</u> your work area.

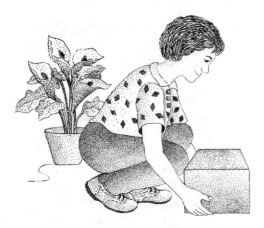

- When you have to move a heavy object, it is better to push it, pull it, or roll it rather than lift and carry it.

- Use your arms to support the object. The muscles of your legs actually do the job of lifting, not the muscles of your back.

- Check your feet before you lift. They should be 12 inches apart to give you a broad base of support and balance.

- Get close to the object being lifted.

- Squat close to the load, grip the object firmly and hold it close to your body. When you want to change direction pivot with your feet, turn your whole body with short steps without twisting your back and neck.

- When you are giving a back rub, making a bed, or moving the patient, work with the direction of your efforts, not against it.

- Avoid twisting your body at the waist. Always turn or pivot completely around.

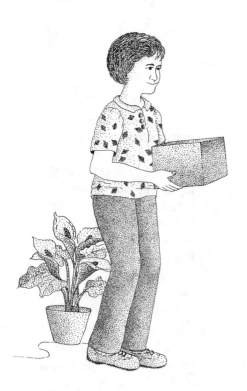

LIFTING & MOVING PATIENTS

A bedridden patient must have his or her position changed often. The patient's body should be straight and properly supported. The correct positioning of the patient's body is referred to as body alignment. Body alignment means the arrangement or adjustment of the patient's body so that all parts of the body are in their proper positions in relation to each other.

Many conditions and injuries make it difficult or even dangerous for a patient to be in a certain position. A pull sheet or lift sheet can help you move the patient in bed more easily. A regular extra sheet folded over many times and placed under the patient can be used as a pull sheet.

When moving the patient, roll, and pull the sheet up tightly on each side next to the patient's body. Grip the rolled portion to slide the patient into the desired position. By using the pull sheet, friction and irritation to the patient's skin are avoided.

Lock Arms With the Patient.

- Have the patient put his arm under your arm (the arm next to him) and behind your shoulder, with his hand over the top of your shoulder. (If you are

standing to the patient's right, his right hand will be on your right shoulder.)

- Put your arm under the patient's arm with your hand on his shoulder.

- On the count of "one, two, three", help the patient pull himself up as you support him. This will raise his head and shoulders.

- To help the patient lie down again, continue supporting him/her with your locked arm and your free hand. Help the patient gently ease back down.

MOVING A PATIENT UP IN BED

- Lock arms with the patient (see above paragraph) and remove the pillow with your free hand. Put the pillow at the top of the bed against the headboard. Put one hand under the patient's shoulder.
- Put your other hand under the patient's buttocks and have the patient bend his knees and place his feet firmly on the mattress.
- Have the patient grasp the headboard. Have your

feet 12 inches apart, bend your knees, and keep your back straight.

- Bend your body from your hips facing the patient and turned slightly toward the head of the bed.
- At the signal, "one, two, three" have the patient pull with his hands toward the head of the bed and push with his feet against the mattress.

- Remove the pillow from the patient's head.

- Slide both your arms under the patient's back to his far shoulder; then slide the patient's shoulders toward you on your arms.

- Slide both your arms as far as you can under the

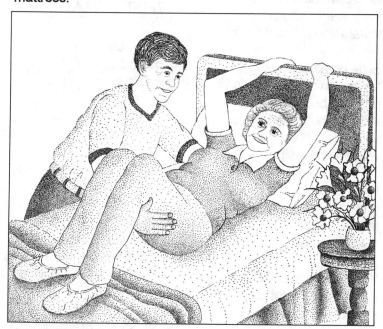

- Lock arms with the patient and put the pillow back in place.

MOVING A HELPLESS PATIENT TO ONE SIDE OF THE BED

patient's buttocks and slide the buttocks toward you. Use a pull sheet whenever possible.

- Keep your knees bent and your back straight as you slide the patient.
- Place both your arms under the patient's lower

legs and slide them toward you on your arms.

ROLLING A PATIENT LIKE A LOG

- Remove the pillow from the patient's head.

- Slide both your arms under the patient's back to his far shoulder; then slide the patient's shoulders toward you on your arms.

- Slide both your arms as far as you can under the patient's buttocks and slide the buttocks towards you. Use a pull sheet whenever possible.

- Place both your arms under the patient's lower legs and slide them toward you on your arms.

- Keep your knees bent and your back straight as you slide the patient.

- Place a pillow between the patient's knees and cross the patient's legs in the direction of movement.

- Keep your knees apart, your back straight and your weight balanced evenly on both feet.

- Roll the patient onto his side like a log, turning his body as a whole unit, without bending his joints. Pull him gently toward you.

MOVING AN AMBULATORY PATIENT FROM THE BED INTO A WHEELCHAIR.

This procedure involves moving a patient who is capable of helping you.

- Place nonslip footwear on the patient's feet.

- If using a medical bed, lower the bed to its lowest horizontal position.

- Position the wheelchair so that the back of the chair is in line with the footboard of the bed.

- Lock the brakes on the wheelchair.

- Raise the footrests of the wheelchair.

- Check the brakes again. Slide both your arms under the patient's back to the far shoulder; then slide

the patient's shoulders
toward you on your arms.

- Slide both arms under the
  patient's buttocks and
  slide the buttocks toward
  you on your arms. Use a
  pull sheet whenever
  possible.

- Slide both your arms
  under the patient's lower
  legs and slide them
  toward you on your arms.

- Keep your knees bent and
  your back straight as you
  slide the patient.

- Slide your arms under the
  patient's arms and on the
  count of three lift the
  patient up.

- Slide the patient's legs
  over the bed.

- Place the patient's arms
  around your shoulders. On
  the count of three, lift,
  pivot the patient around
  and sit the patient in the
  chair.

CHAPTER VII:
OBJECTIVE OBSERVATIONS: SIGNS AND SYMPTOMS

Get into the habit of observing the patient during all your daily contacts. These include: the bedbath, bed making, meal times, and any other quiet time you may be with the patient.

Observing means more than just careful watching. It includes listening and talking to the patient and asking questions. Be alert to changes in a patient's condition or anything unusual that occurs whenever you are with them. Keeping a daily log is a very efficient way of monitoring the patient's physical and mental status on a daily basis. These observations should include:

- You can see some signs of change in a patient's condition. By using your eyes, you can observe a skin rash, reddened areas, or swelling (edema).

- You can feel some signs with your fingers: a change in the patient's pulse rate, puffiness in the skin, dampness (perspiration).

- You can hear some signs, such as a cough or wheezing sounds, when the patient breathes.

- You can smell some signs, such as an odor on a patient's breath.

- Listen to the patient talking for other changes in his or her condition.

THINGS TO OBSERVE IN A PATIENT

Learning how to make useful observations is one of the most important things you will do for your patient. The process of observation never ends, and you learn by doing.

- <u>General appearance</u>. Has this changed?

- <u>Mental condition or mood.</u> Does the patient talk a lot? Very little? Does he talk about the future or the past? Does he talk about where he or she hurts? Is the patient anxious and worried? Calm or very excited? Is the patient talking sensibly or not making sense?

Does the patient appear confused or disoriented? Speaking rapidly? Slowly? Is the patient cooperative? Uncooperative? Belligerent or aggravated?

- Position. Does the patient lie still or does she toss around? Does she like to lie in one position better than others? Does she prefer being on her back? Or on her side? Is she able to move easily?

- Eating and Drinking Habits Does the patient have a healthy appetite? Does he dislike his diet? How much does the patient eat? Is the patient always thirsty or does he drink very little water? Does the patient refuse to eat?

- Sleeping Habits. Is the patient able to sleep? Is he restless? Does the patient sleep more than normal? Is he constantly asleep?

- Skin. Is the patient's skin unusually pale? Is it flushed (red)? Is the skin dry or moist? Are the lips and fingernails turning blue?(cyanotic) Is there any swelling (edema) noticeable? Are there reddened areas? Puffiness? Is the skin shiny? Is the skin cold and clammy? Is it hot?

- Eyes, Ears, Nose and Mouth Does the patient complain that he sees spots or flashes before his eyes? Does bright light bother him? Are his eyes red? is it hard for him to breath through his nose? Is there a mucous discharge from the nose? Does the patient complain that he has a bad taste in his mouth? Is there an odor on his breath? Is the patient able to hear you?

- Breathing. Does the patient wheeze? Does she make other noises when she breathes? Does she cough? Does she cough up sputum and how much? What is the color?Is it bloody? Does she have difficulty breathing or shortness of breath?

- Abdomen, Bowels, & Bladder Does the patient's stomach appear to be distended? Does he complain of gas, belching, or vomitus? Does it contain red blood? Does it look like coffee grounds? Is the patient constipated? How often does he have a bowel movement? What is the color and consistency (hard,soft) of feces(stool)? Is there any blood, or clumps of mucus, or pieces of white material in the feces? How often does the patient urinate? How much does he urinate each time? Is there pain during urination or difficulty to start to urinate? Is there blood in the urine? Is there a peculiar odor or color? Is the patient unable to control his bowels or urine?

- Pain. Where is the pain? How long does the patient say he has had it? Is it constant? Does it come and go? Is the pain dull, sharp, aching or knifelike? Has the patient had medicine for the pain? Did the medicine relieve the pain?

- Daily Activities
  Does the patient dress herself? Does she walk without help? Does she avoid walking altogether?

- Personal Care
  Without help, does the patient brush her teeth? Comb her hair? Go to the bathroom? Wash her face?

- Movements. Is the patient shaking(having tremors or spasms)? Are the patient's movements uncontrollable?

SUBJECTIVE OBSERVATIONS: *SIGNS AND SYMPTOMS*

- Subjective observations are signs and symptoms that can be felt and described only by the patient. Examples are pain, nausea, dizziness, ringing in the ears or headache.

Be sure to take note of these observations and write them down in your daily log for future reference. (See Appendix C)

CHAPTER VIII:
<u>INFECTION CONTROL</u>

A germ is a microorganism. Micro means very small. Germs can be seen only under a microscope. Organism means a living thing. Different kinds of microorganisms (also called microbes) are:

- Viruses
- Bacteria
- Fungi, including molds and yeasts
- Protozoa

Some microorganisms are helpful to people. For example certain microbes cause a chemical change in food called fermentation. Fermentation is the change that produces cottage cheese from milk, beer from grains and cider from apples.

Other kinds of microorganisms, however, are harmful to humans. These microbes cause disease and infection and are called <u>pathogens</u>. They grow best at body temperature, 98.6° F Pathogens destroy human tissue by using it as food. They also give off waste products, called toxins, that are absorbed into and poison the body.

Microbes each have their own natural habitat. When organisms gain access to areas of the body in which they do not belong they become <u>pathogens.</u>

A <u>virus</u> is another type of microorganism. Viruses are much smaller than bacteria, and they cause many of our diseases such as measles, AIDS, and influenza. A French scientist named Louis Pasteur made two important discoveries about bacteria. First, he discovered that many diseases are caused by bacteria. Second, he discovered that bacteria could be killed by heat.

<u>Asepsis</u> means preventing the conditions that allow pathogens to live, multiply, and spread. If germs are not killed, they spread infection and disease from one person to another. Therefore, it is necessary to apply the principles of asepsis in order to prevent germs from spreading. Some ways in which microorganisms are spread are:

- <u>Direct Contact</u>. Touching the patient, rubbing or bathing. Secretions from patient. Urine or feces from the patient.

- <u>Droplet Spread within Three Feet</u>. Sneezing. Coughing.Talking.

- <u>Indirect Contact</u>. Touching objects: Dishes.Bed Linen. Clothing.Belongings.

- <u>Airborne Transmission</u>. Dust particles and moisture in the air.

- <u>Vehicle.</u> Contaminated: Food. Drugs. Water or Blood.

UNIVERSAL PRECAUTIONS

- Gloves must be worn when contact with blood, or body fluids (urine,feces,etc.) is likely.

- Mask and protective eyewear or face shield should be worn during procedures that are likely to generate droplets of body fluids or blood or when the patient is coughing excessively.

- Hand Washing is only effective when:

1. You use enough soap to produce a lather.

2. You rub skin against skin to creation <u>friction</u>, which helps to eliminate microorganisms.

3. You rinse from the clean to the dirty parts of your hands. Rinse with running water from 2 inches above the wrists to the hands and then to the fingertips.

- Take soap from a dispenser, if possible, rather than using a soap dish. Bar soap sits in a pool of soapy water in the soap dish, which is considered contaminated.

- Never use the patient's soap for yourself.

- Hand Washing: Hands must be washed before gloving and after gloves are removed.

- Hand washing must be done before and after direct patient contact, and after handling any of a patient's belongings.

- Home Health Care Providers who have open cuts, sores, or dermatitis on their hands must wear gloves for all patient contact.

<u>CLEAN AND DIRTY</u>. The words clean and dirty have a special meaning.
Clean means uncontaminated. It refers to those articles and places that have not come into contact with pathogens. *Dirty* means contaminated. A used food tray left in a room is dirty and can spread disease. The floor is heavily contaminated. Discard or put in a laundry bag any item that falls to the floor.

CHAPTER IX: <u>BED MAKING</u>

Patients spend most of their time in bed. Some patients are unable to get out of bed easily. As a result, many patients, eat, bathe, and use a bedpan in bed. It is important to make the patient's bed with care and avoid wrinkles. Wrinkles are uncomfortable and restrict the patient's circulation and can cause skin breakdown (decubitus ulcers, or bed sores).

RULES TO FOLLOW: <u>BED MAKING</u>

- Do not shake the bed linen. Shaking spreads germs to everything and everyone in the room, including <u>you</u>.

- Never allow any linen to touch your clothing.

- The bottom sheet must be firm, tight and smooth under the patient's skin. Make sure it is <u>wrinkle free.</u>

- The cotton <u>draw sheet</u> is about half the size of a regular sheet. When a draw sheet is not available, a large sheet can be folded in half widthwise. The fold must always be placed toward the head of the bed.

- Plastic should never touch a patient's skin. If using a plastic draw sheet, be sure to cover it with a cotton sheet.

- Bottom of the bed refers to the mattress pad.

- Top of the bed refers to the top sheet, blanket, and bedspread.

- Remember, you save time and energy by first making as much of the bed as possible on one side before going to the other.

PROCEDURE:
<u>Making the empty bed.</u>

- Stack the bed making linen items on a chair near the bed in the order that you will use them. First things to be used on top, last things to be used on the bottom.

- Pull the mattress to the head of the bed until it touches the headboard.

- Place the mattress pad on the mattress even with the head edge of the mattress.

- Fold the bottom sheet lengthwise and place it on the bed:

A. Place the center fold of the sheet in the center of the mattress from head to foot.

B. Put the small hem at the foot of the bed, even with the edge of the mattress.

C. Place the large hem to the head of the bed.

- Open the sheet. It should now hang evenly the same distance over each side of the bed. The rough edges of the hem should face down toward the mattress and away from the patient.

- Tuck the sheet under the mattress from head to foot. Start at the head and pull toward the foot of the bed as you tuck.

- Stand and work entirely on one side of the bed until that side is finished.

- Fold the draw sheet in half and place it 14 inches down from the head of the bed. Tuck it in. Be sure each piece of linen is straight and even as you tuck.

- Fold the top sheet lengthwise and place it on the bed Repeat the previous directions

for the bottom sheet. DO NOT tuck in at the sides of the bed.

- Repeat for blanket and bedspread, remembering not to tuck them in at the sides of the bed.

PROCEDURE: Making the occupied bed.

The most important part of making an occupied bed is to get the sheets smooth and tight under the patient so that there will be no wrinkles to rub against the patient's skin.

Your job will be easier if you divided the bed in two parts—the side the patient is lying on and the side you are making, so that the weight of the patient is never on the side where you are working.

Usually the occupied bed is made after giving the patient a bed bath. The patient should be covered with the bath blanket while you are making the bed.

Assemble your equipment and place on a chair in the order in which you will use them.

- Loosen all the sheets around the entire bed.

- Remove the bedspread and blanket and fold them over the

back of the chair leaving the patient covered with the top sheet.

- Cover the patient with the bath blanket and ask the patient to hold it. Without exposing the patient, remove the top sheet from under the bath blanket.

- Move or turn the patient to the far side of the bed. Fold the bottom sheet and draw sheet towards the patient's back.
- Raise the plastic draw sheet (if it is clean) over the bath blanket. This strips your side of the bed down to the mattress.

- Take the large clean sheet and fold it in half lengthwise. Do not permit the sheet to touch the floor or your clothing.

- Place it on the bed still folded, with the fold running along the middle of the mattress. Fold the top half of the sheet toward the patient and tuck the folds against his or her back.

- Pull the plastic draw sheet toward you, over the clean bottom sheet and tuck in under the mattress.

- Place the clean cotton draw sheet over the plastic sheet

folded in half. Fold the top half toward the patient, tucking the folds under his or her back as you did with the bottom sheet.

- Go to the opposite side of the bed and roll the patient over the "hump" onto the clean sheets away from you.

- Remove the old bottom sheet and cotton draw sheet from the bed and place in laundry bag being careful not to shake the linen or let it touch your clothing.

- Pull the fresh bottom sheet toward the edge of the bed and tuck it under the mattress from the head to the foot, pulling firmly to remove any wrinkles.

- Pull the draw sheet toward you and tuck under the mattress. (cont....)

- Spread the clean top sheet over the bath blanket with the wide hem to the top. The middle of the sheet should run along the middle of the bed. Remove the bath blanket.

- Tuck the clean top sheet under the mattress at the foot of the bed. Do not tuck in at the sides.

- Spread the blanket and bedspread in the same way.

CHAPTER X:
FEEDING THE PATIENT:

PROCEDURE:
Preparing the patient for a meal.

Eating properly is always important but especially so when a person is ill.

Therapeutic diets are usually ordered by a doctor for patients who cannot be on a regular diet. For example, a patient who has a disorder of the digestive tract may be on a soft or high fiber diet. A diabetic may be on a diet in which total calories are limited along with protein, fat and carbohydrates. A patient suffering from heart disease may be restricted to a low–salt or salt free diet.

A poor appetite does not necessarily mean the body's need for food is lowered. When a person is ill, the body is in a weakened condition and needs as much food as ever, if not more, to return to health. The sight and aroma of food often trigger a person's hunger. The surroundings and the food preparation itself should be as cheerful, appetizing and attractive as possible.

People tend to eat the foods they like. If possible, prepare food that a patient asks for (and is permitted to have). Mealtime is regarded as something to look forward to, especially for the convalescing patient or a patient who is not extremely sick. It is a break in the often boring routine.

Eating in a pleasant atmosphere helps you enjoy and digest your food. Be sure the room is clean, quiet, and odor free. Take away items that might spoil the patient's appetite–urine, bedpan, etc.

- Have the patient wash his hands before eating.

- Raise the backrest so the patient is in a sitting position. If the patient wants to sit in a chair, help him into a robe and slippers and then help him out of bed into a chair.

- Put the tray on the overbed table and adjust it to a comfortable height for the patient.

- If the patient seems to be weak, you might offer to spread the napkin on his lap, or spread the butter on the bread. Cut up the food and pour coffee and drinks if you have to. Remember, the more a patient can do himself the better.

- If the patient decides they are suddenly not hungry, remove the tray and keep the food warm until he is ready to eat.

- Always observe how much the patient has eaten and how much they have had to drink. Did they eat all the food? Half the food? Did the patient eat very little? Eat nothing?

- Record this information separately for breakfast, lunch and dinner on an activity flow sheet (See Appendix C).

- Remove the tray when finished and help the patient sitting in a chair back into bed.

- If the patient ate in bed, brush crumbs from the bed, and straighten and smooth out the sheets.

PROCEDURE: Feeding The Patient Who Is Unable To Feed Himself.

It is difficult for an adult to accept the idea of not being able to feed himself. Try to remain friendly and cheerful especially if the patient seems resentful and depressed.

When helping to feed a patient, it is important not to rush him through the meal. Give the patient ample time to chew his food. Remember, if he didn't need your help, he would be feeding himself.

- Pull up a chair alongside the bed for you to sit in.

- Tuck a napkin under the patient's chin.

- It is easier to feed using a spoon. Fill the spoon half-full and offer to the patient from the tip of the spoon not from the side.

- Try to put the food in one side of the patient's mouth so he can chew it more easily.

- If a patient is paralyzed on one side be sure to feed him on the side that is not paralyzed.

- If the patient cannot see the food, name each mouthful of food as you offer it.

- Offer the foods in a logical order just as you would eat them: soup or juice before the main course.

- Alternate liquids with solids or follow the patient's suggestions on how he would like to eat.

- Always warn the patient if you are offering her something hot or cold. Use a straw for liquids.

- There is no rush. Feed the patient slowly and allow plenty of time between mouthfuls.

- At the end of the meal, note how much food the patient has eaten and how much she has had to drink and note this information in your daily activities log. (see Appendix C)

- Be sure to brush crumbs off the bed and smooth down the sheets.

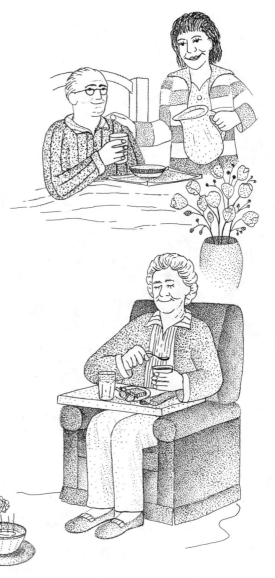

CHAPTER XI: BATHING

Bathing the patient is important for several reasons. Bathing gets rid of dirt. It eliminates body odors and cools the patient. It also stimulates circulation and helps to prevent skin breakdown.

Bathing requires movements of certain body parts: the patient's legs and arms must be lifted and the body turned. This exercises muscles that might otherwise remain unused. During the bathing procedure, observe the patient for unusual body changes: skin rashes, pressure ulcers or reddened areas.

There are four types of baths that may be given, depending on the patient's condition. They are:

Complete bed bath is
given when the patient is too weak or sick to help you. A patient ordered to *complete bed rest* would not be permitted to do anything, especially bathe.

Partial bed bath is given
when a patient is able to care of most of his or her bathing needs. The home care helper would bath areas that are hard to reach, the back or feet.

Tub bath. This bath might
be ordered for therapeutic reasons.

Shower. Showers are given
to patients who have been deemed strong enough to get out of bed and walk around.

SOME POINTS TO REMEMBER WHEN BATHING:

- Usually the complete bed bath is given as part of the morning care routine. After the bath, the occupied bed is made, gown changed, etc.

- Clear off the bedside table and put the items you will be using on it: Soap and soap dish, washcloth, wash basin, face and bath towels, talcum power, clean gown, bath blanket.

- Move the patient close to you so you can work

- without straining your back. Cover the patient with a bath blanket.

- Remember to use good body mechanics: keep your feet separated, stand firmly, bend at your knees and keep your back straight.

- Make a mitten for your hand out of the washcloth to prevent it from dragging across the patient's skin.

- Change the water during the bed bath when it becomes soapy, dirty or cold. Change the water before washing the patient's legs, before washing the back and before washing the genital area.

- Wash one body part at a time. Wash, rinse, and dry each area carefully. Soap has a drying effect on the skin so be sure to rinse off completely.

- Keep the soap in the soap dish so the water does not get too soapy.

- Observe the patient's skin looking for any rashes, redness and tender areas or broken skin.

PROCEDURE: BATHING THE PATIENT

- Remove the bedspread and regular blanket off the bed.

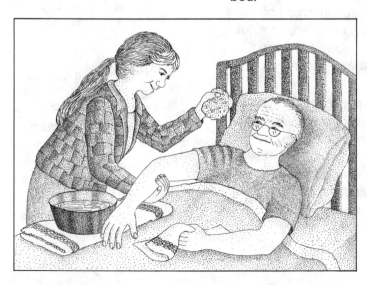

- Remove the patient's gown and jewelry, keeping them covered with the bath blanket.

- Wash the patient's eyes from the nose to the outside of the face. Wash the face carefully if using soap.

- Put a towel lengthwise under the patient's arm to keep the bed from getting wet. Then wash the shoulder, armpit and arm. Use firm, circular strokes. Rinse and dry.

- Place the wash basin on the towel and put the patient's hand in the water. Wash, rinse and dry the hand, and shoulder closest to you.

- Place a towel across the patient's chest and fold the bath blanket down to the abdomen area. Wash and rinse the patient's ears, neck and chest.

- Cover the patient's entire chest with a towel and fold the bath blanket down to the pubic area. Wash the patient's abdomen, navel and any creases in the patient's skin. Dry the area and pull the bath blanket over the abdomen and chest and remove the towels.

- *Empty the dirty water and fill with clean.*

- Remove the bath blanket from the patient's right leg only and place a towel lengthwise under that leg and foot.

- Bend the knee and wash, rinse and dry the leg and foot. If the patient can bend his knee, put the wash basin on the towel and place the patient's foot directly in the water.

- Observe the toenails and skin between the toes for redness and cracking of the skin.

- Dry the patient's leg and foot and between the toes and remove the towel. Cover area with bath blanket.

- Repeat the entire procedure for the other leg and foot. Empty the dirty water, fill with clean.

- Ask the patient to turn on his side with the back towards you.

- Put the towel lengthwise on the bottom sheet near the patient's back. Wash, rinse, and dry the back, buttocks and back of the neck behind the ears. Rub warmed lotion on the back and give the patient a back rub for at least a minute and a half. Look for red areas near the bony areas, hips, elbows. Dry the patient's back, remove the towel and turn him over on his back.

- Empty dirty water and fill with clean. Put on disposable gloves and wash the genital area. Dry well.

- Put a clean gown on the patient.Remove the bedspread and regular blanket off the bed.

PROCEDURE:THE PARTIAL BED BATH

- Place the bath blanket over the patient. Remove the top sheet from under the bath blanket.

- Allow the patient to wash the areas she can easily reach. When finished, empty the dirty water and fill with clean.

- Wash the areas of the body that the patient was unable to reach using the same procedure listed above for the complete bed bath.

- Put a clean gown on the patient and assist them out of bed into a chair.

- Make the empty bed (See Chapter IX)

PROCEDURE: THE TUB BATH

Assemble your equipment on a chair near the bathtub:

Bath towels
Washcloths
Soap
Wash basin
Chair (Placed near the tub)
Clean Gown.
Disinfectant solution

- Wash the bathtub with the disinfectant solution (Before you get the patient up)

- Help the patient out of bed and into a bathrobe and slippers. The patient should either be in a wheelchair or walking with your assistance to the bathtub.

- Place a towel in the bathtub for the patient to sit on.

- Place a towel or bath mat on the floor where the patient will step out of the tub.

- Assist the patient in getting undressed and into the bathtub.

- Help the patient wash himself if help is requested.

The skin of bedridden patients requires special care because of the pressure caused by the bedclothes and the lack of movement. A back rub stimulates circulation, and relaxes the muscles. A good time to do this is during morning care, and after the patient's bath.

PROCEDURE: THE SHOWER

Assemble your equipment on a chair near the shower:(See Tub Bath).

- Help the patient out of bed and into their bathrobe and nonslip slippers.

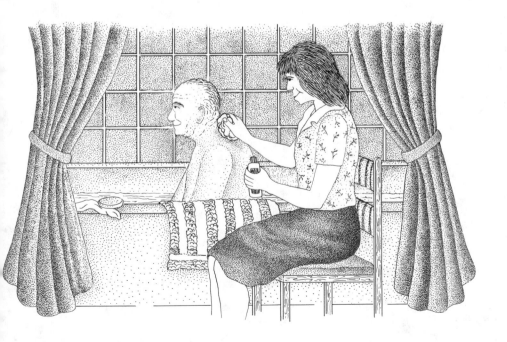

- As an added safety feature, remove all electrical appliances from the room.

- Place a towel on the floor

- Turn on the shower and adjust the water temperature.

- Assist the patient into the shower and hand the patient soap and a wash cloth.

- Place a clean towel on the chair.

- When the patient is finished, turn off the water and assist the patient out of the shower into the chair.

- Help to dry the patient with the towel and assist in putting on pajamas, nightgown, etc. Return the patient to her bed.

PROCEDURE: GIVING A BACK RUB

- Apply lotion to the entire back area, using firm, long strokes from the buttocks to the shoulders and back of neck.

- Use firm pressure and work your stroke upward from the buttocks toward the shoulder.

- Pour a small amount of lotion in your hands and rub together using friction to warm the lotion.

- Use gentle pressure when youstroke downward from the shoulders to the buttocks.

- Concentrate on the bony areas and use a circular motion. Continue for approximately 2 to 3 minutes.

- Pat the patient's back dry and retie the gown.

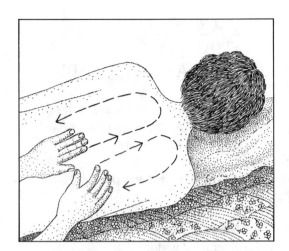

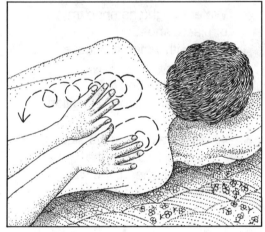

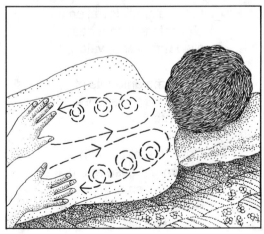

PROCEDURE: SHAMPOOING THE PATIENT'S HAIR.

If the patient is confined to the bed, a shampoo must also be done there.

Assemble your equipment:
Plastic cup
Chair
Basin of water
Pitcher of water
Water trough(shampoo tray) or plastic sheet.
Pillow with waterproof case

- Raise the bed to its highest horizontal position

- Place a chair at the side of the bed close to the patient's head. the chair should be lower than the mattress.

- Place a small towel on the chair along with a basin filled with warm water.

- Put some amounts of cotton in the patient's ears for protection.

- Cover the pillow with a waterproof case and place under the small of the patient's back. The head should be tilted back.

- Place a disposable bed protector on the mattress under the patient's head and place the shampoo trough on top of that.

- A trough can be made by rolling over the three sides of a plastic sheet, making a channel for the water to run off.Put the end of the channel under the patient's head with the open end hanging over the side of the bed into the large basin on the chair.

- Loosen the patient's gown at the neck and lay a washcloth over her eyes.

- Brush the hair downward and fill the cup with water and pour it over the hair until completely wet.

- Apply small amount of shampoo and wash the hair and massage the patient's scalp with your fingertips. Avoid using fingernails.

- Rinse the soap off by pouring water from the cup over the hair.

- Dry the patient's face completely and remove the cotton from the ears.

- Raise the patient's head and wrap the hair with the towel to remove as much moisture as possible.

- Part the patient's hair down the middle to make it easier to comb. Leave a towel spread over the pillow under the head until the hair is completely dry.

It may be difficult for the patient to raise his arms in order to brush or comb his hair. But it's worth the effort:keeping up with personal hygiene always helps a patient to feel better about himself.

- Brush or comb carefully and gently, combing small amounts of hair at a time.

- If the patient cannot sit up in bed or lift their head, separate the hair into small sections and comb each section separately, using a downward motion.Turning the patient's head from side to side will enable you to comb the entire head.

Shaving the Patient's Beard

A regular morning activity for most men is shaving their beard, using either an electric shaver or a razor.

- Raise the head of the bed.

- Spread a small hand towel under the patient's chin. Make sure any dentures are in the mouth.

- Apply warm water or use a damp, warm washcloth on the patient's face to soften the beard.

- Apply shaving cream generously to the face if using a razor.

- Hold the skin taut with one hand as you shave in the direction that the hairs grow. Start under the sideburns and work downward over the cheeks. Work upward on the neck under the chin, using short, firm strokes.

- Rinse the safety razor often.

- Take special care under the nose and around the

lips for these are sensitive areas.

- Wash off the remaining soap, clean your equipment and put it in its proper place.

- Apply aftershave lotion if requested.

CHAPTER XII: BODY ELIMINATION & CLEANSING ENEMAS

When the patient is unable to get out of bed, the urinal and bedpan are used. The urinal is a container the male patient urinates into. The bedpan is a pan which is used by male and female patients to defecate in. Wear disposable gloves whenever you are handling a urinal or bedpan.

Always cover the bedpan and remove it from the patient to the bathroom as quickly as possible after use. If a specimen is required, you would take it at this time. You would also measure urine if the patient is measuring input of liquids and output.

PROCEDURE: OFFERI NG THE BEDPAN

- Find a special holding area for the bedpan and always keep it there.

- Warm the bedpan if necessary by running warm water inside and along the outside rim. Dry the outside of the bedpan and put powder on it to decrease fiction.

- Fold the top sheets back and out of the patient's way.

- Raise the patient's gown but keep the lower part of the body covered.

- Have the patient bend his knees,keeping his feet flat on the mattress, and then raise his hips. You can help the patient raise his buttocks by slipping your hand under the lower part of the back.

- Place the bedpan in position with the seat of the bedpan under the buttocks.

- If the patient is unable to lift his buttocks to get on and off the bedpan, turn the patient on his side with his back to you. Put the bedpan against the buttocks and turn the patient onto the bedpan.

- When the patient has signaled he is finished, wash your hands and put on disposable gloves.

- Help the patient raise his hips and remove the bedpan.

- Help the patient if he or she is unable to clean themselves by turning them on their sides. Clean the anal area with toilet tissue.

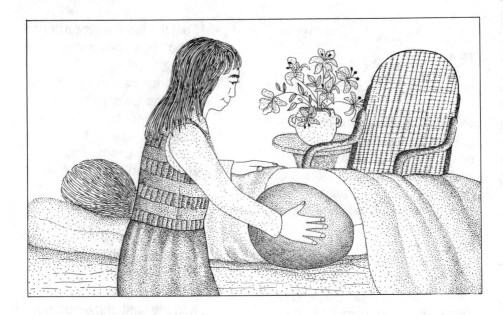

- Cover the bedpan immediately and take it to the bathroom. If a specimen is required, take it now. Observe the feces or urine for abnormal appearance.

- Empty the contents of the bedpan into the toilet. Clean the bedpan with warm, soapy water, dry thoroughly and return it to its holding area.

- Allow the patient to wash his hands in a basin of water.

PROCEDURE: CLEANSING ENEMAS

A cleansing enema is used to wash out waste materials from the lower bowel. Disposable enema kits, which can be purchased at the store, should be used once and then thrown away.

The procedure requires that the patient should lie on his or her left side with the right knee bent up toward the chest. The rectal tube is inserted into the patient's anus.

One third of the enema is given with the patient on his or her left side. Another third is given with the patient lying on his stomach and the remainder is given as the patient lies on the right side. This procedure allows the enema to enter all sections of the colon; descending, transverse and ascending.

If the patient complains of a cramplike pain after the enema has started, stop the flow and then start again when the pain is gone.

- Assemble all your equipment:
  Disposable enema kit
  Bedpan and cover
  Toilet tissue
  Disposable bed protector
  Paper Towel

- Wash your hands and put on gloves.

- Put the disposable bed protector under the patient's buttocks.

- Turn the patient on his left side with the right knee up towards the chest.

- Place the bedpan within easy reach.

- Close the clamp on the enema tubing and fill the enema container with 1000cc of tap water, heated at 105°F.

- If your instructions call for soap-suds enema, add the package of enema soap to the water in the container. Stir gently using the tip of the tubing. Do not create suds.

- Add 2 teaspoons of salt to the water if a saline enema is needed.

- Do not add anything to

tap–water–only enema.

- Open the clamp on the tubing and let some of the solution run into the bedpan. This warms the tube and eliminates air in the tube which can cause flatus.

- Put some lubricating jelly on the enema tip going up the tube 2-4 inches. Make sure the tip is not plugged.

- With the patient on his side, raise the upper buttocks and gently insert the enema tip 2-4 inches. If you feel resistance, stop.

- Hold the enema container 12 inches above the anus and open the clamp. Instruct the patient to take slow, deep breaths to relieve any cramping that may occur.

- A third of the solution is given while the patient is on the left side, a third while on the stomach, and the remainder while lying on the right side.

- After the enema container is almost empty, close the clamp and slowly withdraw the tubing.

- Wrap toilet tissue paper around the tip to avoid

contamination and place it in the enema container.

- The patient should try to hold the solution in as long as possible. Help the patient onto the bedpan. Put the toilet tissue within easy reach.

- Or, you may assist the patient to the bathroom. Stay near for assistance. The patient should not flush the toilet until the results can be observed.

- Observe the color, odor, consistency and amount of the results of the enema, focusing on anything that does not appear to be normal.

- Is the stool hard? Soft? Large in amount? Small in amount? Black in color? Streaked with yellow, red, gray or white? Does it have a bad odor? Look like perked coffee grounds?

- Write all observations down in the daily log.

- Empty, clean and store the bedpan equipment if used.

- Discard the removable bed protector.

- Allow the patient to wash his hands.

- Remove gloves and wash your hands.

Prepackaged, Ready to-Use Enema

The ready-to-use enema is effective and easy to use. Follow the same procedures to prepare the patient. Turn the patient on his left side, and bend the right knee towards the chest. Raise the upper buttocks and gently insert the enema tip, two inches through the anus into the rectum.

- Gently squeeze the plastic bottle until all the liquid goes into the rectum. Remove the tube from the patient's anus.

- Place the empty plastic bottle in the bottle and discard properly.

- The patient should try to hold the solution as long as possible. Help the patient onto the bedpan. Place the toilet tissue within easy reach.

OIL RETENTION ENEMA

When the retention enema is given, the patient is expected to retain the enema solution for 10-20 minutes. These enemas are given to:

- help soften the feces and stimulate evaluation
- Lubricate the inside surface of the lower intestine.
- Ease the passage of feces without straining.
- Provide laxative benefits when oral laxatives cannot be used.
- Soften fecal impaction (hard stools retained in the lower bowel)

CHAPTER XIII: POTENTIAL SKIN PROBLEMS; HOW TO AVOID AND TREAT THEM.

Pressure ulcers (decubitus ulcers) also called bedsores, are areas where the skin has broken down because of prolonged pressure on a part of the body where there is a loss of circulation. Lack of blood flow to the injured area destroys tissues. If bedsores are not treated, they get larger and often become quite painful. They usually occur in places where the bones are close to the body surface: hip bones, shoulder blades, backbone, elbows, knees, heels, sides of ankles, and the back of the head over the ears. The pressure can come from the body lying in one position for too long or from casts or bandages. Even wrinkles in the bed linen can be a cause of bedsores.

Bedsores are often made worse by continued pressure, lack of cleanliness, moisture, and heat. Also, perspiration, urine, feces, wound discharges or soap that has not been thoroughly rinsed off the skin.

Observe the skin for signs of redness, tenderness and heat. A bedsore occurs when the skin is broken. Treatment should be specified by the attending physician. The open wound must be kept clean at all times to prevent infection.

There are special devices available that can reduce the pressure on the bony prominences: sheepskin booties and elbow pads, flotation beds and commode flotation pads. The specialty bed, which constantly turns the patient, is another device to alleviate pressure points.

Patients who are over–weight or obese can develop bedsores where skin touches skin, such as the folds of the buttocks and between the thighs.

PROCEDURE: PREVENTING BEDSORES

- The patient's position in bed should change every 2 hours.

- Bedpans can create and worsen existing bedsores due to friction when moving on and off. The patient should not sit on the bedpan for any longer than is necessary; pressure from sitting on the rim can also create and aggravate bedsores.

- Cleanliness: keep the patient's gown clean and dry.

- Use mild soap when washing the patient's skin and rinse thoroughly.

- Rub tender areas with skin lotion to increase circulation. Rub in a circular motion but not directly on the affected area.

- Use powder or corn starch on areas where skin surfaces come together and form creases: under the breasts of women, between the buttocks and in the folds of skin on the abdoman. Wash the corn starch off completely at bathing time and then reapply.

- When making the bed, check the linen for wrinkles.
- Remove any hard objects from the bed; hair pins, bed crumbs, etc.

- Use a disposable bed protector so any soiled areas can be cleaned easily. Remove the bed protector when it becomes wet. Never allow plastic to touch the patient's skin.

- If the patient wears a disposable diaper, check the skin carefully for a reaction to the material and to irritations caused by urine and feces. Change diapers immediately if they become soiled or wet.

PROCEDURE: PREVENTING ULCERS IN THE INCONTINENT PATIENT

Assemble all your equipment.

Basin of water
Soap
Corn Starch or powder
Towels
Disposable gloves
Lotion
Washcloths
Bedpan

- Roll the patient on his side.

- Put on the disposable gloves.

- Using toilet tissue, wipe away the waste material from the skin. Wash the area that was soiled clean. Dispose of soiled tissue in the bedpan.

- Dry the area with a circular motion to stimulate blood circulation.

- Apply lotion to the buttocks and back and massage as you rub it in.

- Apply powder or corn starch on the surfaces where skin touches skin. (In creases, etc.) Apply lightly, and do not allow any to cake together.

- Leave the top sheets loose so air can flow freely over the patient.

- Turn the patient to a different position every two hours.

- Place all dirty and soiled linen in the laundry bag and remove.

- Remove and discard gloves.

CHAPTER IVX:
ORAL HYGIENE
PROCEDURE:
BRUSHING TEETH

Oral hygiene is the care of the mouth and teeth. At times, a person who is ill will have a bad taste in their mouth due to medications taken. Or the tongue may be covered with a grayish coating that spoils the appetite. Cleaning the patient's mouth and teeth is an essential and very important part of daily patient care.

Assemble your equipment by the bed.

Mouthwash
Fresh water
Disposable cup
Straw
Toothbrush
Toothpaste
Emesis basin
Face Towel

- Wash your hands

- Place the towel across the patient's chest.

- Mix 1/2 cup water with 1/2 cup mouthwash and allow the patient to rinse her mouth. Hold the emesis basin under the chin for the patient.

- Wet the toothbrush and place toothpaste on it. If the patient is able, allow her to brush her own teeth.

- Help the patient to rinse the mouth.

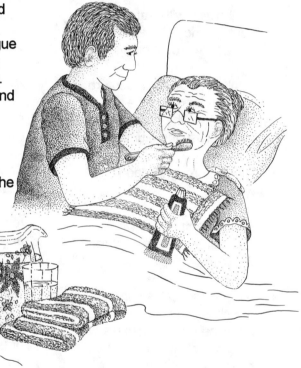

PROCEDURE:
CLEANING THE DENTURES

- Assemble your equipment by the bed.

- Wash your hands.

- Put on disposable gloves.

- Place tissue in the emesis basin.

- Have the patient remove his dentures and place them in the basin.

- Fill the sink with water so the dentures don't break if you accidently drop them.

- Apply toothpaste or denture cleanser and with the dentures in the palm of your hand, brush them until clean.

- Rinse thoroughly under cool water.

- Fill the denture cup with water and salt. Place the dentures in the cup.

- Fill the disposable cup with 1/2 mouthwash and 1/2 water and have the patient rinse his mouth. Hold the basin at the patient's chin.

- Be sure dentures are moist before giving them back to the patient.

- Leave a clean denture cup with a clean solution on the side table within the patient's reach.

CARE OF THE OCULAR PROSTHESIS (ARTIFICIAL EYE)

Cleaning an artificial eye is an important part of daily personal hygiene. Tears and mucus leave deposits on the eye, and a film develops that dulls its' luster. Also, these deposits often irritate the eye socket.

Most daily accumulations can be cleaned without removing the artificial eye from the socket. Daily cleaning can be done in the shower using Johnson's Baby Shampoo. Enzymes in the shampoo break down protein that accumulates on the eye and removes mucus from the eyelids and lashes.

Away from the shower and without removing it, rinse the prosthesis with sterile saline solution. Use a moist cotton swab or gauze, wiping gently towards the nose. Wiping away from the nose might dislodge or rotate the prosthesis.

Artificial tears such as Celluvisc, or oily lubricants, such as Sil-Ophtho or Duratears can help to lessen irritation caused by low tear flow.("dry eyes")

Clean the artificial eye each morning, but remove only

occasionally unless there are special problems. (Contact your doctor or ocularist) Remove it when there are excess secretions. Remember, removal exposes the eye socket to bacteria.

Once the prosthesis is removed for cleaning, it can take three (3) days for the body's natural lubricants to coat the surface of the eye with soothing secretions. During this time you may use artificial tears or other lubricants to reduce irritation.

PROCEDURE: REMOVING THE ARTIFICIAL EYE.

Assemble your equipment by the bed:

An eyecup half willed with warm water.

Gauze strips

Basin filled with lukewarm

Water

Cotton balls

- Wash your hands.

- If the patient is removing or inserting the eyes, allow him to wash his hands.

- The patient should be lying down with his eyes closed. Clean any secretions from the upper eyelid using the cotton balls and warm water. Wipe gently towards the nose using a clean cottonball with each swipe.

- To remove the artificial eye, depress the lower eyelid with your thumb. As you do so, lift the upper lid with your forefinger. The eye should slide out into your hand. Line the bottom of the eyecup with gauze strips.

- Place the eye in the eyecup and let it soak in water.

- Wash the outside of the eye socket with cotton balls and warm water, once again using a clean cotton ball with each swipe.

- Take the eyecup to the bathroom and fill the sink with water.

- Wash the eye in warm running water. Hold it between the tip of the thumb and fingers and gently rub it with diluted baby shampoo. A hard contact lens cleaner or enzymatic cleaner may also be used as a soak.

- Gently dry the eye using a piece of gauze. Place the slightly moistened eye on dry gauze in the eyecup and return to the patient.

To Remove With A Suction Cup:

- tilt the patient's head downward

- have them look up, and press upward with your index finger from the skin below the lower lid.

- Apply the suction cup to the center of the prosthesis.

- Pull it up and out from the lower lid and then down from the upper lid.
- Never try to pull the prosthesis straight out of the socket.

INSERTING THE ARTIFICIAL EYE

- Always wet the artificial eye before inserting it.

- Raise the upper lid with your forefinger. Hold the eye in your free hand between your thumb and index finger

- Insert the upper portion and release the lid.

- Then pull down on the lower lid while pushing up on the prosthesis.

- Push the prosthesis towards the socket to remove air that might be trapped behind the artificial eye.

Note: Some patients can experience socket contraction if the artificial eye is left out for a period of time, even if it is only for overnight.

- If the prosthesis is going to be left out of the socket for any length of time, it should be stored in a sterile saline or balanced salt solution.

- The prosthesis should be professionally cleaned and polished by the ocularist at least once a year. Scratches and deposits that accumulate over a period of time should be removed professionally.

CHAPTER XV: MASSAGE THERAPY AND RANGE OF MOTION

A patient who is unable to get out of bed easily will not be getting the proper exercise. Range of motion exercises move each muscle and joint through its full range of motion.

Active Range of Motion The patient is able to move his limbs through the exercises by himself.

Passive Range of Motion: The patient is unable to do the exercises and requires assistance.

Active Assist Range of Motion: The patient works with the home health care provider but only to the extent that he is able.

- When doing the exercises, follow a logical sequence so each joint and muscle is exercised. One logical choice would be to start with the head and work down towards the feet. Be gentle. Never bend or force a body part farther than it can go.

JOINT ARTICULATION: Passive movement of any joint by rotation or bending.

Joint articulation opens the joints and increases their range of motion. Passive joint articulation implies that the patient does not resist or help. It involves letting go of control of voluntary movements, relaxing and not resisting the external manipulation. If resistance is present, gentle shaking is a good way to get the patient to relax. The joints should never be forced to move, nor should they be moved past what can be tolerated by the patient.

- STRETCHING: Extension of the muscles or body by pulling or bending a body part.

Once again, passive stretching requires that the patient be relaxed and not help with the movement or the manipulation. All general stretches should be applied with the following procedures:

1. Have the patient begin breathing with full, relaxed breaths.
2. Move to the first point of resistance in the stretch.
3. On the next inhale, apply a steady even pressure and move just past the point of resistance.

4. Hold the pressure steady as the patient exhales and releases.
5. Continue to hold an even pressure. Do not give up any slack during the successive inhales. Do not apply more pressure. Never force or bounce the stretch. Do only as far as the patient allows for comfort.
6. When the stretch is complete, wait until the end of an exhale and slowly release the pressure. Maintain the stretch for a minimum of three (3) breaths.
7. Move the body part slowly back to its original resting position.
8. Gently shake or vibrate the area stretched.

DIRECT PRESSURE is one of the most effective neutralizers of chronic pain. It is capable of breaking up knots in tight muscles and stretches the muscles and tendons. It also allows for more independent movement of muscles, increased range of motion and realignment of the body with gravity.

Direct pressure can be applied with the fingertips, thumb, knuckles, and heel of the hand. You can use direct pressure over any knotted muscle. Direct pressure should be applied with the same procedures used on stretching.

When you have determined that the muscle is relaxed, wait until the end of an exhale and then slowly release the pressure. Again, maintain pressure for at least three (3) breathes.

When direct pressure is being used to neutralize a painful area, deep pressure is best maintained for at least seven (7) seconds.

BASIC MASSAGE TECHNIQUES

Massage is the sharing of touch–hands on body, on head, hands or feet. This section will discuss holistic or intuitive massage to distinguish it from Swedish massage. Holistic massage treats the individual as a whole, not just concentrating on physical conditions. Its movements are slower and more meditative. The receiver's role is to be relaxed but alert, while the giver should concentrate on bringing an attitude of genuine caring to the massage.

The basic massage is divided into strokes and parts of the body.

When giving a massage, be sure to ask for feedback on what feels good. The slower and more rhythmical your strokes, the more relaxed and safe the patient will feel.

A good massage benefits the patient on many levels. Physically, its benefits include relaxing and toning muscles and stretching the connective tissue of joints.

On a mental level, massage relieves stress and anxiety. A caring massage creates feelings of well-being, trust and joy.

As you work on each new part of the body, you begin by lightly oiling it. This allows your hands to slide smoothly and evenly without any friction or jerkiness. It also nourishes the skin. Only a thin film is necessary to lubricate the skin. For larger expanses, like the back or hairy areas, you may need to apply extra oil. The oil is rubbed into the skin by using long, gliding strokes.

There is no need to buy ready-made massage oils. You can use vegetable oil, such as sunflower, safflower or coconut. Almond oil is very pleasant but expensive. You can also use mineral oils, such as baby oil, though these are less easily absorbed. If you use a plain oil, try scenting it with a few drops of perfume or essential oils.

Keep your oil in a corked bottle or a flip-top plastic bottle. Holding your hands away from you, pour a little oil in the palm. Rub your palms together to spread the oil equally. Begin to apply the oil by using the long stroke.

FREE STROKING OR GLIDING STROKES

Apply the flat, open palm over an extended portion of the body. Your hands should be open and relaxed as you stroke. The movements are long, continuous and rounded with no breaks in the flow of movement as you change direction.

Free Stroking is particularly relaxing when done with light pressure and slow, even movements.

Heavier pressure can also be applied and is used to enhance the blood and lymph circulation. Heavy pressure can be applied to the back in any direction.

MEDIUM DEPTH STROKES

Kneading works more deeply on the large muscle masses and uses the whole hand to pull and squeeze bunches of flesh- one hand releasing as the other gathers a new handful. Rock smoothly as if you were kneading dough, alternately squeezing and releasing handfuls of flesh in a broad, circular motion. This technique tones the muscles and improves circulation. It is an excellent form of passive exercise.

FOLDING :Scoop your fingers in a half circle in toward the thumb, all the while squeezing and kneading the mucles between them.Lift and Squeeze, then release, one hand after the other.

DEEP TISSUE STROKES

Deep and focused, these friction movements make use of the thumbs, fingertips or heels of hands to reach down into the tissue, penetrating below the superficial muscle layers. Work around the joints with deep tissue strokes. It is important work deeper gradually but you will generally find that the body is less fragile than you think.

HEEL OF HAND PRESSURE: Push the heels of your hand firmly forward into the flesh, bringing one heel down just behind the other.Your hand should move alternately and rhythmically.

ALTERNATE OR CIRCULAR THUMBS: With your fingers relaxed, push with

your thumbs away from you in a circular motion.. As a beginner, don't be daunted by how much there is to learn- practise a little at a time and you will soon find that your hands are relaxed and the strokes come naturally to you.

Return the thumbs to the beginning position with light pressure. Do not be afraid to apply pressure to the muscles. Do not move your thumbs with the whole hand and arm. Keep them flexible so as to allow them to move independently of your hand.

CIRCULAR FINGERTIPS:
Place the pads of your fingertips on the body and gradually work into the muscles, holding your fingers in place.

SKIN ROLLING is done by placing the tips of the thumbs together and then pulling a roll of skin towards them with the fingertips, lifting and squeezing, one or two fingers at a time. A continuous roll is done by reaching out with individual fingers to pull more skin into the roll as the thumbs move. Skin rolling can be done in any direction.

PERCUSSION:
Percussion belongs in its own category, for unlike the other strokes, its movements are stimulating rather than relaxing. It

includes a range of brisk, rhythmic strokes performed repeatedly with alternate hands. The main value of percussion is to stimulate the soft tissue areas, such as thighs and buttocks, toning the skin and improving circulation. Practise the strokes on your own leg first. Your hands should be relaxed and your wrists loose before you start. Experiment with different speeds and pressures. Percussion is not always appropriate. Reserve it for those occasions where a vigorous approach is required.

HACKING: Bounce the sides of your hands alternately and fairly rapidly up and down, palms facing one another and fingers loosely together. Get a good rhythm going before hacking muscles directly.

PUMMELLING: Loosely clench your fists, then repeat the same rhythmic succession of strokes with the fleshy sides of your fists. Your hands should be relaxed so that they bounce firmly yet lightly up and down.

CUPPING: Cup your hands, arching them at the knuckles, fingers straight(like pincers). Repeat the same rapid strokes as hacking and pummelling. Your cupped hands trap air against the skin, then release it, making a loud sucking sound.

THE BASIC MASSAGE SEQUENCE:

Caution: There are certain conditions in which massage is not recommended. These include skin eruptions, such as boils, or infectious rashes; large bruises; varicose veins;fever,inflamed joints;tumour or any undiagnosed lumps; cardiovascular problems, such as thrombosis and phlebitis.And only give massage in cases of arthritis when the inflammation has gone.

1. THE BACK

You start your massage with the back, first working broadly over the whole area, then concentrating on smaller portions in turn: the shoulder blades and upper back;the lower back, buttocks, sides and finally, the spine itself.

2. BACK OF LEGS

Next is the back of the legs. Begin by lightly oiling the hands, then massage each leg. Work your way up the leg then knead your way down. Finally massage the foot.

3. SHOULDERS, NECK AND SCALP

Begin with the shoulders working on both front and back at once. Then, turning the head to one side, work on each shoulder separately. Complete this section by massaging the scalp.

4. FACE
Start at the forehead and work down to the chin. Work outward from the center to the sides.

5. ARMS AND HANDS
Each arm is massaged separately. Just as you did with the legs, first work up the arm, then knead down. End this section by massaging the wrist and hand.

6. FRONT OF TORSO
Focus on the rib-cage and sides of torso. Then move down to circle around the abdomen. Next, work up from the belly in long sweeping strokes.

7. FRONT OF LEGS
Apply oil to both legs, then concentrate on one at a time-working up the leg, circling the kneecap on the way down, then kneading down the leg again. End this section with the feet.

8. ANKLE
Hold the foot firmly with one hand, using your free hand to work around the anklebone with fingers or thumb. Work around the joint with small circling strokes, first on one side, then the other.

8A. ROTATING THE ANKLE
Hold the leg just above the ankle with one hand, grasp the foot with your free hand and slowly move it around in a wide circle, first in one direction for a few turns, then in the opposite direction. Circle the foot to the limits of its flexibility.

The human foot is a highly complex structure consisting of 26 small bones, some of which form two large supporting arches. The feet not only carry the entire weight of the body, they also serve as wonderful shock absorbers. Also, the soles of the feet contain thousand of nerve endings, with reflex connections to the whole of the rest of the body. When you massage the feet, you are affecting the entire body, not just the feet themselves. For this reason, many masseurs concentrate on a foot massage when there is not enough time for a full body massage.

9. THE FOOT:STRETCHING
9A. THE TOES
First, stretch the toes apart, sideways, then stretch each toe backward and forward. Check how far you can stretch the toes with the patient.

9B. CLEANING BETWEEN THE TENDONS
Hold the sole of the foot in one hand, toes pointing upward. Use

the thumb or fingers of your free hand to press slowly along each channel between the tendons that link the base of the ankle to the toes.

9B. THUMBING THE SOLE
Support the foot with one hand. With your freehand, work across the whole of the sole with the thumb, making small, firm, circling strokes. Start at the heel and end at the ball of the foot, just under the toes.

9D. WRINGING THE TOES.
One at a time, hold each toe at the base between your thumb and fingers and tug gently. Twist each toe a little from side to side as your fingers slide to the tip and off.

10. THE SCALP:
The scalp also can get tense which in turn, cause tension headaches and also hair problems such as dandruff and hair loss. Massage can relieve the tension and aid the circulation.

10A: PULLING OFF THE
        HAIR:
Take a bunch of hair and pull gently from the roots, letting the hair slowly slide off your fingers.

10B: ROTATING THE SCALP:
Spread your hand over the head and gently rotate it, moving the scalp against the bone.

10C: SHAMPOOING:
This is a wonderful way to vigorously massage the scalp. Rub all over the scalp with your fingertips.

CHAPTER XVI:
KEEPING A SCHEDULE OF DAILY CARE.

It is important to establish a daily schedule for the patient. It gives them continuity to their day and helps them stay in touch reality. A sample schedule for the day might include:

EARLY MORNING CARE:*BEFORE BREAKFAST*

- Offer the bedpan or urinal

- Using a fresh wash cloth, wash the patient's face and hands.

- Help patient with oral hygiene: cleaning teeth, dentures, etc.

- Tidy up surrounding area. Place fresh drinking water close by.

- Raise the head of the bed. Or offer to help patient to sit up in bed.

- Serve breakfast

MORNING CARE: *AFTER BREAKFAST*

- Offer bedpan or urinal

- Help patient with oral hygiene.

- Bathe the patient. Allowing for the differences in the patient's capabilities, give the patient a complete bed bath, partial bed bath, shower, or tub bath.

- Offer a fresh gown to the patient

- Help the patient shave or comb hair.

- Make the bed: occupied or unoccupied.

- General straightening of the area.

AFTERNOON CARE: *AFTER LUNCH*

- Check patient's gown and change if necessary

- Straighten up surrounding area

- Offer bedpan or urinal or assist to the bathroom.

- Help patient with oral hygiene

- Using clean washcloth, assist patient in washing hands and face.

EVENING CARE: *AFTER DINNER*

- Offer bedpan or urinal

- Wash the patient's hands and face

- Assist with oral hygiene

- Give a back rub

- Change the draw sheet

- offer an extra blanket for bedtime.

- Offer fresh drinking water.

Documentation of all activitites will allow you to keep on top of any changes in the patient's condition, no matter how small or insignificant they may appear to be. Purchase a simple notebook and write brief notes of your care. All caregivers should be required to maintain the notebook and sign off at the end of each day. Remember to be clear, concise, timely and *accurate* about your observations. (See Appendix C)

APPENDIX A: *organizations to contact for help*

ALCOHOL and DRUG ABUSE

ALCOHOLICS ANONYMOUS
PO BOX 459
GRAND CENTRAL STATION
NEW YORK,NY 10163
212-870-3400

   The national office in New York can direct you to a local AA Chapter. AA assists alcoholics to become and remain sober through self help groups.

AL ANON FAMILY GROUPS
1600 Corporate Landing Prkway
Virginia Beach, VA 23454
757-563-1600

   This organization helps family members and friends of alcoholics to cope.. They also make referrels and will send out brochures on how alcoholism affects families

NATIONAL CLEARING HOUSE
for ALCOHOL and DRUG
INFORMATION
PO BOX 2345
ROCKVILLE, MD 20847-2345
800-729-6686

   This organization has publications on alcoholism and drug use with a focus on prevention. There are materials on treatment as well.

ALZHEIMER'S DISEASE

ALZHEIMER'S ASSOCIATION
919 N. MICHIGAN AVE.
SUITE 1000
CHICAGO, IL. 60611
800-272-3900

   Also known as the Alzheimer's Disease and Related Disorders Association, this organization provides information and referrals to local chapters. The local chapter will direct people to local services and support groups that are available.

ALZHEIMER'S DISEASE
EDUCATION and REFERRAL
CENTER
P.O. BOX 8250
SILVER SPRING, MD 20907-8250
800-438-4380

   This organization is directed by the National Institute on Aging and has information on all aspects of Alzheimer's Disease.

NATIONAL INSTITUTE of
NEUROLOGICAL DISORDERS
and STROKE
Information Office

Building 31, Room 8A16
31 Center Drive., MSC2540
Bethesda,MD 20892-2540
800-352-9424
    This office is part of the
National Institutes of Health and
has information about stroke and
other brain disorders, such as
Parkinson's, Alzheimer's and
epilepsy.

ARTHRITIS AND OSTEOPOROSIS

ARTHRITIS FOUNDATION
INFORMATION LINE
P.O. BOX 19000
ATLANTA,GA 30326
800-283-7800
    This organization provides
information and makes referrels to
local chapters that in turn support
groups, events and classes.

NATIONAL ARTHRITIS and
MUSCULOSKELETAL and SKIN
DISEASES INFORMATION
CLEARINGHOUSE
1 AMS CIRCLE
BETHESDA,MD 20892
301-495-4484
    This is a federal clearinghouse
that has publications covering a
host of disorders and diseases
that affect bones, joints and skin.

NATIONAL OSTEOPOROSIS
FOUNDATION
1150 17th. St. N.W. Suite 500
Washington, DC 20036
800-223-9994

202-223-2226
    This organization will send out
material relating to the causes,
prevention, and treatment of
osteoporosis.

CANCER

AMERICAN CANCER SOCIETY
1599 Clifton Rd. NE
Atlanta, GA 30329
800-227-2345
404-320-3333
    This organization answers
questions that deal with cancer
detection, treatment and current
research . They will also refer
callers to local chapters for more
information on local services.

CANCER INFORMATION
SERVICE
National Cancer Institute
Building 31, Room 10A24
Bethesda, MD 20892
800-422-6237
    This organization offers a
helpline that provides information
on topics such as detection of
cancer and treatment to financial
help and home care. It also refers
callers to local organizations,
cancer centers and support
groups.

NATIONAL COALITION for
CANCER SURVIVORSHIP
1010 Wayne Ave
Silver Spring, MD 20910
301-650-8868

This is a private, nonprofit organization that offers information on cancer treatments, costs, insurance coverage and employment. It also refers people diagnosed with cancer to support groups.

CAREGIVER SERVICES

AGING NETWORK SERVICES
4400 East West Hwy
Suite 907
Bethesda, MD 20814
301-657-4329
This is a private business. For a fee they will refer you to a geriatrric care manager in your parent's area. The manager serves as a liaison for the family and will coordinate services for your parent.

AMERICAN ASSOCIATION of RETIRED PERSONS (AARP)
601 E. St. , NW
Washington, DC 20049
202-434-2277
800-424-3410
AARP offers brochures on caregiver stress, how to care from a distance and a variety of other issues that face the elderly and their families. Most of these are free.

CHILDREN OF AGING PARENTS (CAPS)
1609 Woodbourne Rd., Suite 302A
Levittown, PA 19057

215-945-6900
800-227-7294
This organization provides information on cargiving and refers callers to support groups and other resources. They charge a small fee for brochures and copies of articles from the group's newsletters, which costs $20 a year for six issues.

ELDERCARE LOCATOR
800-677-1116
This organization is run by the National Association of Area Agencies on Aging and is a good place to start your search for local services. A helpline is at your service to guide you in reaching the area agency on aging located in your paren'ts hometown.

NATIONAL ASSOCIATION OF PROFESSIONAL GERIATRIC CARE MANAGERS
1604 North Country Club Rd.
Tucson, AZ 85716
520-881-8008
This is a trade association for care managers. They also make referrals to geriatric care managers.

NATIONAL ASSOCIATION OF SOCIAL WORKERS
750 First St., N.E.
Washington, DC 20002
800-638-8799
This is a trade association for social workers. They also give

referrals to local social workers who serve a dual function as care managers or therapists.

NATIONAL FEDERATION OF INTERFAITH VOLUNTEER CAREGIVERS
368 Broadway, Suite 103
Kingston, NY12401
800-350-7438
914-331-1358

This private, nonprofit group administers over 400 regional offices that send volunteers into the homes of people who need care, company and supervision.

WELL SPOUSE FOUNDATION
610 Lexington Ave, #814
New York, NY 10022
212-644-1241

This organization offers emotional support to husbands and wifes caring for a sick spouse. Members are directed to support groups and receive a newsletter six times a year.

DEATH AND DYING

CHOICE IN DYING
200 Varick St.
New York, NY 10014
212-366-5540
800-989-9455

This organization provides information along with legal forms that include a living will and

durable power of attorney for health care that are up-to-date and specific to each state. Counseling is available from staff lawyers, nurses and social workers.

FUNERAL & MEMORIAL SOCIETIES OF AMERICA
P.O. Box 10
Hinesburg,VT. 05461
800-765-0107

This organization offers guidance on how to plan inexpensive and dignified funerals and memorial services.

HEMLOCK SOCIETY USA
P.O. Box 101810
Denver, CO 80250
800-247-7421

This organiation promotes the right to euthanasia- refusal of life-saving treatments and physician-assisted suicide. Telephone counseling is available along with referrals to local chapters.

NATIONAL FUNERAL DIRECTORS ASSOCIATION
11121 West Oklahoma Ave
Milwaukee, WI 53227
414-541-2500
800-228-6332

This organization offers guidance in locating a funeral director, and planning memorial services.

NATIONAL RIGHT TO LIFE
COMMITTEE
419 Seventh St., NW, Suite 500
Washington, DC 20004
202-626-8800
   This organization opposes
abortion and euthanasia. They
have drafted a "Will to Live" form
which states a person's wishes to
be kept on life suport regardless
of the medical prognosis. They will
also help people seeking medical
treatment that a doctor or hospital
refuses to provide.

DIABETES

AMERICAN ASSOCIATION OF
DIABETES EDUCATORS
444 N. Michigan Ave.Ste. 1240
Chicago, Il. 60611
800-338-3633
   This is a professional
association for diabetes
educators-health workers trained
and certified to teach diabetics
how to manage the disease. The
Association offers referrals to local
diabetes educators.

AMERICAN DIABETES
ASSOCIATION
1660 Duke St.
Alexandria, VA 22314
800-232-3472
   This organization provides
information on diabetes, from
medical treatment to financial
concerns. They will also direct you

to state chapters for referrals to
local doctors and support groups.

NATIONAL DIABETES
INFORMATION
CLEARINGHOUSE
1 Information Way
Bethesda, MD 20892
301-654-3327
   This clearinghouse sends out
information on all aspects of
diabetes. They are sponsored by
the National Institute of Diabetes
and Digestive and Kidney
Disease.s.

DIGESTIVE DISEASES

NATIONAL DIGESTIVE
DISEASES INFORMATION
CLEARINGHOUSE
2 Information Way
Bethesda, MD 20892
301-654-3810
800-891-5389
   This clearinghouse sends out
brochures, scientific articles and
other data on digestive diseases,
from indigestion to ulcers and
gallstones.

DRIVING

AAA FOUNDATION FOR
TRAFFIC SAFETY
1440 New York Ave., NW
Suite 201
Washington, DC 20005
800-305-7233

202-638-5944

This organization offers pamphlets, and videos on driving and safety. A booklet aimed at older drives is available containing a self-exam to test knowledge and skills, and information about a flexibility training program.

NATIONAL SAFETY COUNCIL
1121 Spring Lake Dr.
Itasca, Il. 60143
800-621-6244

This Council offers a course for elderly drivers called "Coaching the Mature Drive." Call for more information.

EXERCISE

AMERICAN ALLIANCE FOR HEALTH,PHYSICAL EDUCATION, RECREATION and DANCE.
P.O. Box 385
Oxon Hills, MD 20750
800-321-0789

The Alliance publishes books on exercise and other physical activities, including books for the elderly and the disabled.

AMERICAN PHYSICAL THERAPY ASSOCIATION
1111 North Fairfax St.
Alexandria, VA 22314
703-684-2782

The APTA has a pamphlet on exercise tips for the elderly.

ARTHRITIS FOUNDATION
P.O. Box 19000
Atlanta,GA 30326
800-283-7800

The Foundaton offers information on exercise and rehabilitation . They also make referrals to local chapters.

PRESIDENT'S COUNCIL on PHYSICAL FITNESS and SPORTS
200 Independence Ave S.W. #738-H
Washington, DC 20201
202-690-9000

The Council provides information on physical fitness and exercise programs. Available is the "Nolan Ryan Fitness Guide" for people over 40. For a copy, write to: Nolan Ryan Fitness Guide, P.O. Box 22091, Albany,NY 12201-2091

FINANCES

INTERNATIONAL ASSOCIATION FOR FINANCIAL PLANNING
Two Concourse Parkway,Suite 800
Atlanta, GA 30328
800-945-4237
404-395-1605

This trade association has material on hiring a planner and offers referrals to local financial planners.

NATIONAL FOUNDATION for
CONSUMER CREDIT
8611 Second Ave., Suite 100
Silver Spring,MD 20910
800-388-2227
   This Foundation makes
referrals to local Consumer Credit
Counseling Service offices, which
will provide free or low-cost
counseling on budgeting and debt
management.

PENSION RIGHTS CENTER
918 16th. St., NW, Suite 704
Washington, DC 20006-2902
202-296-3776
   This center provides
consumers with legal guidance
and other pertinant information.

SOCIAL SECURITY
ADMINISTRATION
800-772-1213
   Call this number to arrange for
direct deposit of social security
checks, to notify the agency of a
change of address, check benefits
or for general information on
social security.

GENERAL LISTINGS

AMERICAN ASSOCIATION of
RETIRED PERSONS
601 E. St., NW
Washington, DC 20049
202-434-2277
800-424-3410
   AARP is one of the largest
lobbying and educational
organzations in the country. It

offers free booklets on a wide
range of topics, such as housing
options, home care, and
caregiver stress. There are also
money-saving programs for
members; a travel service and
mail order pharmacy, volunteer
programs and services. Call to
find out about local chapters and
membership benefits.

CONSUMER INFORMATION
CENTER
"Catalog"
Pueblo, CO 81009
719-948-3334
   This is a federal agency that
distributes more than 200
consumer publications from
various departments and
agencies of the government.
Topics listed are: health, nutrition,
insurance and aging. Write to the
above address for a catalogue of
publications. Most are free or cost
less than a dollar.

NATIONAL ASSOCIATION OF
AREA AGENCIES ON AGING.
(NAAAA)
 1112 16th. St.,NW, Suite 100
Washington, DC 20036
   This is a private, nonprofit
organization that runs an
Eldercare Locator (800-677-1116)
which directs people to local
agencies on aging.

NATIONAL COUNCIL on the
AGING

409 Third St.,SW
Washington, DC 20024
202-479-1200

This is a private, nonprofit organization which initiates programs, trains professionals and advocates on behalf of the elderly. The NCOA has specialized membership units for professionals and volunteers including the National Institute of Senior Centers, the National Institute of Senior Housing and the National Institute on Financial Issues and Services for Elders.The NCOA makes referrals to local services and has information available on caregiving and related topics.

NATIONAL COUNCIL of SENIOR CITIZENS
1331 F. St., NW
Washington, DC 20004
202-347-8800

This is a membership organization-a smaller version of AARP- that advocates for the elderly in Washington, DC. They offer members benefits such as group insurance, low-priced prescription drugs and travel services.

NATIONAL INSTITUTE on AGING INFORMATION CENTER
P.O. Box 8057
Gaithersburg,MD 20898
800-222-2225

This is a division of the National Institutes of Health that supports research on aging and health. It produces several free publications, including dozens of "Age Pages" which deal with information on geriatric health issues.

HOME CARE

NATIONAL ASSOCIATION for HOME CARE
228 7th. St. S.E.
Washington, DC 20003
202-547-7424

This organization represents a wide range of home-care organizations. On request, it will send out a pamphlet of tips on choosing a home-care agency.

VISITING NURSE ASSOCIATIONS of AMERICA
3801 East Florida Ave., Suite 900
Denver, CO 80210
800-426-2547

The VNAA represents nearly 500 visiting nurse associations across the country which offer skilled nursing care, therapy, hospice care, counseling, home health aides and homemakers, nutrition counseling and chore service.

HOSPICE

HOSPICE ASSOCIATION of AMERICA
228 7th. St. S.E.
Washington, DC 20003
202-546-4759

This trade association is part of the National Asociation of Home Care. They make referrals to local hospices and offers information on hospice care.

HOSPICE HELPLINE
NATIONAL HOSPICE
ORGANIZATION
1901 N. Moore St., Suite 901
Arlington, VA 22209
800-658-8898

The National Hospice Organization represents hospices nationwide. Through its Helpline, it provides information about hospice care and makes referrals to local hospices.

HOUSING

AMERICAN ASSOCIATION of HOMES and SERVICES for the AGING
901 E. St., NW, Suite 500
Washington, DC 20004
202-783-2242

This Association offers consumer brochures on various housing options, nursing homes and community services. It also publishes the *Consumer's Directory of Continueing Care Retirement Communities* which lists and describes more than 550 retirement communities.

ASSISTED LIVING FEDERATION of AMERICA
9411 Lee Highway

Plaza Suite J
Fairfax, VA 22031
703-691-8100

This is a professional association that offers a couple of helpful brochures on assisted living and what to look for when choosing an assisted living home.

NATIONAL SHARED HOUSING
RESOURCE CENTER
321 East 25th. St.
Baltimore, MD 21218
410-235-4454

This organization offers information about shared housing and makes referrals to local organizations that help bring together roommates.

NURSING HOMES

NATIONAL CITIZENS'
COALITION for NURSING HOME
REFORM
1424 16th. St. ,NW, Suite 202
Washington, DC 20036
202-332-2275

This coalition consists of advocacy organizations, ombudsman programs and individuals working to improve nursing home care. It offers guidance in selecting a nursing home and procedures in filing complaints.

WOMEN'S SERVICES
OLDER WOMEN'S LEAGUE
666 11th. St., NW, Suite 700
Washington, DC 20001
800-825-3695

This is a grass roots organization advocating for economic and social equity of midlife and older women. It offers fact sheets on issues such as pensions, women's health and caregiving, and also provides some referrals. Requests should be made in writing, accompanied by a self-addressed, stamped envelope

APPENDIX B

SAMPLE FORMS FOR BACKGROUND CHECKS & FINGERPRINTING

GUIDELINES FOR FINGERPRINT CARD SUBMISSION

The National Child Protection Act was passed by Congress as a mandate for states to pass legislation that would enable citizens to do criminal background checks on people they were going to hire for child care or elder care. It is impossible to list all the different procedures for background checks for each state. However, you may contact the Department of Justice in your state to find out the guidelines. The following information on fingerprints is for residents of California only.

ELDER CARE EMPLOYERS (Section 15660 Welfare and
                        Institutions Code)

The Bureau of Criminal Identification and Information (BCII) provides State summary criminal history information to employers of persons who are unlicensed and providing non–medical domestic or personal care to an aged or disabled adult in the adult's own home. This also includes applicant's for in–home supportive services or personal care services under the Medi–Cal program administered by individual county agencies pursuant to Section 15660 of the Welfare and Institutions Code. As defined:

- "Elder" means any person who resides in a state, 65 years of age or older.

- "Dependent Adult" means any person residing in a state between the ages of 18 and 64, who has physical or mental limitations which restrict his or her ability to carry out normal activities or protect his or her own rights.

PROCEDURE FOR SUBMISSION (California only. For all other states contact the Department of Justice in your area)

Please submit a completed 10 print Applicant Fingerprint Card (BID-7. Each request must be accompanied by a $32 processing fee. Checks or money orders should be made payable to Department of Justice. For an additional $10 fee, you may take advantage of an optional, expedite service which offers a 17 working day turnaround for the (D.O.J.) State response only.

RELEASE OF INFORMATION

Welfare and Institutions Code 15660 limits the criminal history information which can be released. Under this Section, you will only receive information on the following:

- Arrests for specified sex offenses against a minor, sexual battery, willful cruelty to a child, inflicting injury upon a child, cruelty to an elder or dependent adult, theft, robbery,burglary or any felony offense.

- Arrests for specified offenses that have resulted in conviction or indicate active prosecution.

Criminal record information for specified offenses will only be released if the arrest occurred within 10 years of the date of the employer's request.

AUTHORIZATION TO RELEASE INFORMATION

TO WHOM IT MAY CONCERN:

Having made application for employment with _____,
I hereby authorize any representative of said person, bearing this release or a copy of it, to obtain any information in your files pertaining to my employment, preemployment, military, arrest, conviction, driving, credit or education history, including but not limited to, academic achievement, attendance, athletic performance, personal history, performance reports, background investigations, and polygraph examination results.

I hereby release you, as the custodian of such records, and any law enforcement or criminal justice agency, school, college, university, or other educational institution, hospital or other repository of medical records, credit bureau, lending institution, consumer reporting agency, or retail business establishment including its officers, employees, or related personnel both individually and collectively from any and all liability for damage of whatever kind, which may at any time result to me, my heirs, family or associates because of compliance with this authorization and request to release information, or any attempt to comply with it. Should there be any questions as to the validity of this release, you may contact me as indicated below.

A photocopy of this release form will be valid as an original thereof, even though the said photocopy does not contain an original writing of my signature.

I understand that I have the right to receive a copy of this authorization and acknowledge that I have received copy of it.

_____   _____
Signature   Date

_____   _____
Full Name(Please Print)   SS # **

_____
Current Address

** In accordance with the federal privacy act of 1974, disclosure of the S.S. N. is voluntary. The S.S.N. will be used only for identification purposes to ensure that proper records are obtained.

APPENDIX C

SCHEDULE OF DAILY CARE LOG SHEET

Date			
DIET`	Breakfast	Lunch	Dinner
Ate all food			
Ate 1/2 food			
Refused to eat			
Comments			

Procedures	Date/Time	Date/Time	Date/Time
Oral Hygiene			
Bed Bath			
Partial Bed Bath			
Tub			
Back Rub			
Linens Changed			

Elimination	Appearance	Color	Consistency	Amount
Bowel Move-ment				
Involuntary B.M.				
Urinated				
Incontinent				
Constipated				
Comments				

Activity	Date/Time			
Bed Rest				
Up In Chair				
Up In Room				
Walking				
Range-of-Motion	Rotating	Bending		
Joints				
Arms				
Legs				
Ankle				
Comments				

INDEX

ORDER FORM
Call Toll Free and order NOW!

1-800-617-7667
916-987-1378 (fax)

Postal Orders: Creative Opportunities
P.O. Box 2461
Orangevale, CA 95662

Please send the books to:

Company Name_____

Name: _____

Address:_____

City: _____

Telephone: _____

Cost of Book $9.95ea.
*Sales Tax: _____
**Shipping: Book rate: _____

*Please add 7.75% for books shipped to California addresses.
**$2.00 for the first book and 75 cents for each additional book. (Surface shipping may take three to four weeks)
Air Mail: $3.50 per book.

Payment: : Check or Money Order to :
Creative Opportunities